REA's Interactive
Flashcards®

NCLEX-RN®

National Council Licensure
Examination for Registered Nurses

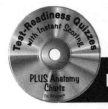

Premium Edition with CD-ROM

Marion Brandis, RN
Barbara Fomenko Harrah, RN, MSN
...ski, RN, MS, CS-ANP

D1113313

Research & Education Association
Visit our website at
www.rea.com

The information contained herein presents scenarios and other narrative consistent with targeted preparation for the NCLEX-RN Exam. The book's contents are deemed to be accurate and relevant to the cited subject matter at the time of publication. Neither the publisher, Research & Education Association, Inc., nor the author(s) is engaged in nor shall be construed as offering legal, nursing or medical advice or assistance or a plan of care. If legal, nursing or medical assistance is required, the services of a competent professional person should be sought.

NCLEX-RN® is a registered trademark of the National Council of State Boards of Nursing, Inc.

Research & Education Association
61 Ethel Road West
Piscataway, New Jersey 08854
E-mail: info@rea.com

REA's Interactive Flashcards® NCLEX-RN® (National Council Licensure Examination for Registered Nurses) Premium Edition with CD-ROM

Printed in the United States of America

Library of Congress Control Number 2008928749

ISBN-13: 978-0-7386-0460-2
ISBN-10: 0-7386-0460-7

H08-0101

About This Premium Edition with CD-ROM

REA's unique interactive flashcard book with CD-ROM will help you succeed on the NCLEX-RN exam so you can be licensed in your exciting and rewarding career as a Registered Nurse.

With this flashcard book you won't have to deal with an awkward box and its hundreds of loose cards. Here, it's all bound neatly inside, with questions on one side, a place to write your response, and the answers and explanations on the flip side. It is portable and useful in many ways — for quick study, rapid review, and easy reference.

In this **Premium Edition with CD-ROM**, we've made it easy for you to hone your study skills. As you go through the book, look for the STOP sign. When you see it, pause your study and take one of the **four test-readiness quizzes on CD**. This will test how well you know the material up to that point. It's an excellent way to build knowledge and confidence. When done, move ahead until you reach the next STOP sign.

Also included on the CD are four invaluable reference charts that you can return to time and again: **Anatomy & Physiology**; **The Skeletal System**; **The Muscular System**; and **Circulatory System**.

We are proud of this one-of-a-kind versatile flashcard book, and we hope you find it valuable in your quest to become a Registered Nurse.

Larry B. Kling
Chief Editor

Test-Readiness Quizzes on CD
After studying questions 1 through 86, take Quiz 1.
Take Quiz 2 after studying questions 87 through 170.
After studying questions 171 through 258, take Quiz 3.
Quiz 4 starts after question 343.

Questions

Q1

The nurse is aware that the priority intervention for the client hospitalized for clinical depression is:

1) encouraging the client's expression of emotions
2) encouraging the client to obtain exercise
3) removing harmful objects from the client's room
4) allowing the client to sleep as much as possible

*Your Own Answer*_____

Q2

Clients at greatest potential risk for suicide include:

1) adolescents and the elderly
2) persons with chronic illnesses and/or pain
3) alcohol and drug abusers
4) all of the above

*Your Own Answer*_____

Q3

All of the following are potential indicators of risk for suicide except:

1) being male, < 19 or > 45 years old
2) previous suicide attempt(s)
3) being a cigarette smoker
4) decreased social support

*Your Own Answer*_____

Correct Answers

A1

Answer 3 is correct as the priority nursing intervention is always client safety. It is essential to keep harmful objects out of the reach of a depressed client, who may think about or attempt suicide or self-mutilation. While the clinically depressed client does need encouragement to express his or her feelings and obtain exercise, these are not the first priorities of care; therefore, answers 1 and 2 are incorrect. Although sleep disturbance (too much or too little) is a common symptom of clinical depression, treatment would not include allowing for unlimited sleep; therefore, answer 4 is not correct.

A2

The correct answer is 4. Suicide is most often accomplished by people fitting into at least one of these three categories listed in answers 1, 2, and 3.

A3

The correct answer is 3. Smoking cigarettes has not been associated with a potential for either depression or suicide risk. The other indicators, answers 1, 2, and 4, are in fact serious risk factors for a potential suicide attempt.

Questions

The nurse is aware that the hospitalized depressed client will need all of the following EXCEPT:

1) a full schedule of outside visitors
2) assistance in decision making
3) frequent or constant observation
4) participation in group discussions

*Your Own Answer*_____

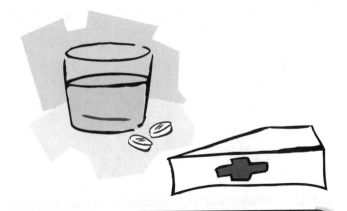

The nurse is aware that the usual therapeutic adult dose at the beginning of treatment and time of onset for the antidepressant medication fluoxetine (Prozac) is:

1) 50 mg/day and 1-2 weeks for effective onset
2) 20 mg/day and 1-4 weeks for effective onset
3) 40 mg/day and 1-4 weeks for effective onset
4) 20 mg/day and 4-6 weeks for effective onset

*Your Own Answer*_____

Correct Answers

A4

Symptoms of depression include social withdrawal, difficulty with decision making, and suicidal ideation or attempts. The nurse should provide the client with, or arrange for the client to have, those interventions listed in answers 2, 3, and 4, above. Therefore, answer 1 is correct; for safety reasons, it is essential to monitor and restrict visitors from outside the unit, who may leave behind objects that the client could later use in self-harm.

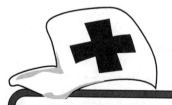

A5

Answer 2 is correct. The dose may be increased by 20-mg increments, but only after several weeks to first determine the efficacy of the starting dose. Answers 1, 3, and 4 are therefore incorrect: 40 and 50 mgs would not be starting doses for fluoxetene, due to the possibility of unpleasant side effects; 1–2 weeks is not long enough and 4-6 weeks is longer than necessary to determine the drug's efficacy.

Questions

Q6

When caring for the depressed client, the nurse expects to assess for which of the following symptoms and behaviors?

1) fearfulness, avoidance, pounding heart, chills or hot flushes, trembling
2) repetitive behaviors (e.g., handwashing) or mental acts (e.g., silent word repetition)
3) hopelessness, despair, psychomotor retardation, slowed speech and thought processes
4) irritability, aggression, psychomotor agitation, flight of ideas, grandiosity
5) catatonia, aggression, agitation, grimacing

②

*Your Own Answer*_____

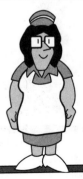

Q7

The physician orders the MAOI tranylcypromine (Parnate) for a client. The nurse is aware that the client should be assessed for:

1) tachycardia and vomiting
2) muscular rigidity and drooling
3) excessive thirst or dry mouth
4) convulsions

*Your Own Answer*_____

Correct Answers

Answer 3 is correct; these are some of the persistent symptoms of clinical depression. Answer 1 outlines some of the symptoms associated with panic attacks; the physiological symptoms are particularly unique to this form of severe anxiety disorder. Answer 2 is incorrect; the behaviors listed are characteristic of compulsive disorder. Answer 4 is not the best choice; these symptoms are typical of a manic episode seen with bipolar disorder. Answer 5 describes the symptoms of schizophrenia; although this organic brain disorder shares some of the symptoms of bipolar disorder, it is distinguished by severe physiological symptoms, such as catatonia and facial grimacing.

Answer 1 is correct; tachycardia and vomiting, along with headache and palpitations, may indicate a hypertensive crisis, a common adverse effect requiring immediate physician notification. Muscular rigidity and drooling are some of the extrapyramidal side effects associated with Haldol. Excessive thirst is a common side effect of the tricyclic antidepressants and of Haldol. Convulsions occur only with an overdose of this drug. Therefore, answers 2, 3, and 4 are incorrect.

Questions

Q8

A new client is admitted to the psychiatric unit. The nurse's intake interview will include the client's report of which of the following:

1) changes in sleep pattern, weight, appetite, and bowel function
2) occupation, marital status, education, and religion
3) presenting problem, or reason the client is seeking help
4) all of the above

3

*Your Own Answer*_____

Q9

A client on a psychiatric floor refuses to take the medication prescribed for him. The nurse, wishing to maintain her trusting relationship with this client, should:

1) hide the medicine in the client's food at each meal in order to avoid a confrontation
2) give the medication at the same times each day to build trust with the client
3) let the client decide when and where to take the medication to indicate growing trust
4) call the security team to forcibly medicate the client, showing who is in charge

4

*Your Own Answer*_____

Correct Answers

A8

Answer 4 is correct; the nurse would be interested in assessing somatic changes (answer 1) the client's general history (answer 2), and the presenting problem in the client's own words (answer 3).

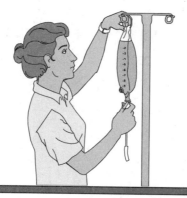

A9

Psychiatric clients are often fearful, anxious, and untrusting. Answer 1 would constitute tricking the client, which, if discovered would destroy any trust already established; therefore, this method is not best. Answer 3 is incorrect; the time and place for giving medication is not realistically up to the client and indicates a lack of professional responsibility. Answer 4 is unnecessary and would be destructive of the therapeutic trusting relationship already established. Therefore, answer 2 is the best choice; consistency of time of giving medication may enhance the trusting, therapeutic relationship between the client and nurse.

Questions

A nurse in a community clinic assesses every client for psychiatric disorders. The most important initial primary prevention intervention she can offer is:

1) an opportunity for the client to discuss home-life and job concerns
2) psychopharmacologic treatment through a referral to a psychiatrist
3) membership in an ongoing, twice-weekly behavioral therapy group
4) assessment of vital signs, weight, height, and laboratory values

*Your Own Answer*_____

A client on a psychiatric unit who has slept only 3 hours for the past four nights is rapidly pacing the hallways, muttering vulgar words to himself, occasionally yelling out that he is the president of the United States, and expressing irritability toward the nurse who is encouraging him to join the other patients for dinner. This client is suffering from:

1) schizophrenia and paranoia
2) a manic phase of bipolar disorder
3) a depressive phase of bipolar disorder
4) clinical depression with suicidal intent

*Your Own Answer*_____

Correct Answers

A10

Answers 2 and 3 are both incorrect; they are not primary prevention interventions, and would be relevant only to the client with an already established psychiatric diagnosis. Answer 4, while relevant to many nursing assessments, is not the most important initial assessment intervention for a potential psychiatric disorder, such as depression. Answer 1 is correct, demonstrating primary prevention through assessment for risk factors —stress and role conflict at home and work—for mental/emotional illness.

A11

These behaviors—vulgar speech, hyperactivity, decreased need for sleep, delusions, and possibly weight loss—are typical to the manic phase of bipolar disorder; therefore, answer 2 is correct. Schizophrenia and paranoia (answer 1), may include withdrawal, negativism, religiosity, and especially auditory hallucinations. The depressive phase of bipolar disorder, along with clinical depression, also may include decreased appetite and insomnia, but are further characterized by fatigue, dysphoric mood, and movement retardation; therefore, answers 3 and 4 are incorrect.

Questions

The nurse is leading the biweekly therapy and psychoeducation session on an in-patient psychiatric floor. She knows that in order to establish a safe, therapeutic environment for all of the clients, it is important to:

1) set up a contract outlining the nurse's expectations for limits on behavior during and between sessions
2) allow the group members to speak freely and for as long as they wish at all times in group sessions
3) encourage the group members to speak privately among themselves about the session between group meetings
4) encourage the members of the group, with the nurse's guidance, to set agreed-upon parameters for behavior during and between sessions

Your Own Answer

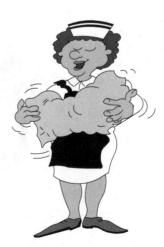

Correct Answers

Answer 1, not the best choice, indicates the nurse's concern for limit setting and enforcement of appropriate behavior, but is not likely to be of therapeutic benefit to psychiatric patients. Answer 2, also incorrect, shows lack of responsibility for limit-setting on the part of the nurse. Answer 3 shows the nurse's lack of understanding of the importance of encouraging trust between the clients during *and* outside the sessions; therefore, this is not a good choice. Only answer 4, the correct choice, indicates the nurse's understanding of the importance of both limit-setting and self-efficacy to creating an environment of trust and safety amongst group members.

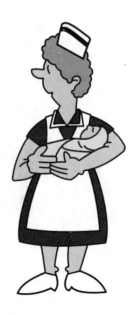

Questions

Q13

A client is admitted to an in-patient psychiatric unit. The nurse performs an intake interview and discovers that the client hears voices telling her to set fire to all her possessions to rid them of germs; cannot tolerate the sight and smell of many of her past favorite foods; thinks that she is Mary Magdalene; and likes to curl up in a chair and rock back and forth when she feels frightened. The nurse is aware that this client is most likely suffering from:

1) schizophrenia
2) depression
3) Down's syndrome
4) borderline personality

*Your Own Answer*_____

Q14

The eating disorder known as anorexia nervosa is characterized by:

1) recurrent binge eating and an accompanying fear of not being able to stop eating voluntarily
2) intense fear of becoming fat, an unrealistic body image, and weight decrease of at least 25%
3) nervous shaking of the hands and trembling of the mouth at the sight, smell, and taste of all food
4) persistent eating of nonnutritive substances, such as chalk or laundry starch, for a period of at least one month

*Your Own Answer*_____

Correct Answers

A13

Answer 1 is correct: auditory hallucinations, delusions, hypersensitivity to sights and smells, and autistic movements are the classic symptoms of schizophrenia. Other than delusions in borderline personality, none of these other symptoms is specifically present in depression, Down's syndrome, or borderline personality; therefore, answers 2, 3, and 4 are incorrect.

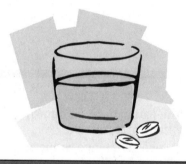

A14

Answer 1 describes the eating disorder known as bulimia, and is therefore incorrect. Answer 3 is not a description of any known medical disorder, and is incorrect. Answer 4 is characteristic of pica and is not the correct choice. Answer 2 is correct; it describes some of the symptoms of anorexia nervosa, a serious condition with no underlying physical cause, which can, however, be fatal.

Questions

Q15

Down's syndrome is most often characterized by which of the following physical traits?

1) hypertonic muscles; long, thick eyelashes; large nose with protruding bridge; long narrow neck; and enlarged genitalia
2) hypotonic muscles; short, sparse eyelashes; high-set, large ears; sunken abdomen; and small genitalia
3) hypotonic muscles; short, stubby fingers; small head with a flattened face; protruding abdomen; and small genitalia
4) hypertonic muscles; large, high-set ears; small nose with depressed bridge; large head with rounded face; and small genitalia

*Your Own Answer*_____

Q16

Hallucinations, a common symptom of schizophrenia, are defined as:

1) sensory impressions—hearing voices, seeing visions, or having tactile experiences—in the absence of external stimuli
2) actual stimuli that is misinterpreted; for example, thinking that a person who is hailing a cab is aiming a gun at you
3) fixed beliefs, which are false, such as believing oneself to be Jesus Christ or the president of the United States
4) recurring nightmares, over the course of two weeks or longer, in which evil spirits and demons are pursuing you relentlessly

*Your Own Answer*_____

Correct Answers

A15

Only answer 3 correctly describes the classic appearance of a person with the congenital anomaly called Down's syndrome. Other characteristics include sparse hair, arched palate and protruding tongue, and mental retardation with developmental delays. Therefore, answers 1, 2, and 4 are incorrect.

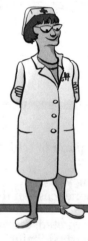

A16

Answer 2 defines illusions, while answer 3 defines delusions; therefore they are both incorrect. Answer 4 is not a particular clinical diagnosis, and is also incorrect. Answer 1 correctly gives the definition for hallucinations, one of the most disturbing symptoms for one suffering from schizophrenia.

Questions

(9)

Q17

The defense mechanism known as rationalization is defined as:

1) use of excessive reasoning or logic to avoid the experience of and responsibility for otherwise disturbing feelings or thoughts
2) offering of a logical or socially acceptable explanation to justify otherwise unacceptable feelings or behavior
3) unconscious exclusion from conscious awareness of conflictive or painful thoughts, feelings, or memories
4) shift of emotions from the object or person to whom it was originally directed to one less emotionally dangerous

*Your Own Answer*_____

Q18

Which of the following examples involves sexual abuse?

1) Two 21-year-old college students agree to engage in sexual activity after attending a campus fraternity party.
2) A secretary's boss pats her bottom, tells her "dirty" jokes, and repeatedly pressures her to go on a date with him when they are at work.
3) A 45-year-old man initiates sexual activity with his 8-year-old niece, and threatens to hurt her if she tells on him.
4) A man forcefully initiates sexual activity with his wife of 20 years after she clearly expresses her desire to go to sleep.

*Your Own Answer*_____

Correct Answers

A17

Answer 1 defines the defense mechanism known as intellectualization, answer 3 defines repression, and answer 4 defines displacement; these are therefore incorrect. Answer 2, the correct choice, defines the process of rationalization.

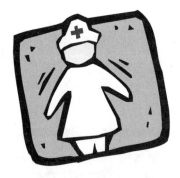

A18

Answer 3 is correct; sexual abuse is an inappropriate expression of power by an adult, not necessarily a relative, through sexual activity with a child who cannot comprehend or consent freely in this activity. It often involves secrecy as well. Answer 1, incorrect, is an example of consensual sex between two adults. Answer 2 is an example of sexual harrassment in the workplace. In answer 4, sexual assault is occurring between two adults.

Questions

Q19

A 20-year-old female college student reports to the nurse that she eats dinner most nights in her dormitory's dining hall, after which she goes back to her room and, if she is alone, consumes an extra sandwich, 6 or 7 doughnuts, a bowl of ice cream, and 4 or 5 candy bars. She is aware that this pattern of eating is unhealthy, yet she feels convinced that she cannot control these eating binges. Following these binges, she induces vomiting. Often her mood becomes depressed after these episodes. The nurse realizes that the student is suffering from

1) anorexia nervosa
2) pica
3) generalized anxiety
4) bulimia

*Your Own Answer*_____

Q20

Some of the presenting signs and symptoms of alcohol abuse include the following:

1) relaxation, euphoria, impaired judgment, slurred speech, detachment from reality
2) depressed mood, impaired concentration, motor ataxia, increased reaction time
3) relaxation, mild euphoria, reduced inhibition, red eyes, dry mouth, increased appetite
4) sudden rush of euphoria, agitation, diaphoresis, insomnia, increased energy

*Your Own Answer*_____

Correct Answers

A19

Answer 4 is correct; bulimia is one of the most common eating disorders that strikes girls usually in adolescence and can continue untreated due to its secretive nature. Anorexia nervosa, also seen most often in young women, is characterized by self-starvation due to an unrealistic perception of the body as overweight; therefore, answer 1 is not correct. Pica is a disorder involving the craving for nonnutritive substances such as dirt, clay, or laundry starch; answer 2 is therefore incorrect. Generalized anxiety disorders do not necessarily involve compulsive eating as the focus for behavior; therefore, answer 3 is incorrect.

A20

Answer 1 lists some of the signs and symptoms of heroin abuse; answer 3 presents the signs and symptoms of marijuana abuse, and answer 4 lists signs and symptoms for cocaine abuse. These are therefore all incorrect. Answer 2, which is correct, is a list of some of the signs and symptoms of persistent alcohol abuse, which further includes problems with hand-eye coordination; decreased REM sleep; and depression of cognition, memory, and affect.

Questions

The progression and recovery of the alcoholic include the following steps in which order?

I.   defeat by alcoholism is admitted and honest desire for help is expressed
II. healthy level of self-esteem and contentment with sobriety
III. surreptitious drinking and increase in alcohol tolerance
IV. impaired cognition and obsession with drinking

1) II, I, IV, III
2) IV, III, II, I
3) I, II, III, IV
4) III, IV, I, II

*Your Own Answer*_____

A 65-year-old client has just undergone an above-the-ankle amputation for a diabetes-related complication. The nurse will expect the client to display the following feelings and behaviors in which order?

I.   denial and regression
II. acceptance and adaptation
Ill. mourning the loss and focus on strengths
IV. guilt, anger, and discouragement

1) IV, III, I, II
2) II, IV, III, I
3) IV, I, III, II
4) I, II, III, IV

*Your Own Answer*_____

Correct Answers

The correct answer is 4; this is the correct order of some of the steps in the progression from chronic alcoholism to rehabilitation and recovery. Answers 1, 2, and 3 are therefore incorrect.

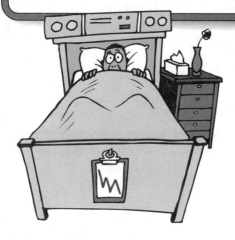

Similar to the stages of acceptance of impending death, alterations of body image bring a progression of attitude and behavior changes. Answer 3 correctly lists the order of progression for an adult coming to terms with the loss of a body part. Therefore, answers 1, 2, and 4 are incorrect.

Questions

Q23

The priority nursing intervention for a cancer patient receiving chemotherapy postoperatively is:

1) counselling for altered body image
2) maintenance of nutritional regimen
3) rest and respite for other caregivers
4) comfort through positioning, pain meds, etc.

*Your Own Answer*_____

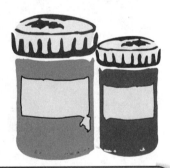

Q24

The hospital is holding an educational session about cancer. The nurse-educator mentions all of the following early warning signs of cancer EXCEPT:

1) change in bowel or bladder habits
2) decrease in sleep from 8 to 6 hours
3) a lesion that does not heal
4) obvious change in a wart or mole

*Your Own Answer*_____

Correct Answers

A23

Maintaining the comfort of the postoperative cancer patient through positioning and pain management is the priority nursing intervention; therefore, answer 4 is correct. Providing emotional support and encouraging the client's nutritional intake, answers 1 and 2, are important as well, but not the top priority of care. The well-being of other caregivers indirectly affects this client, and is not the priority intervention; therefore, answer 3 is not the best choice.

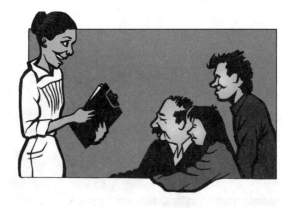

A24

Answers 1, 3, and 4 list some of the many early warning signs of cancer. A decrease in the need for sleep, especially as we age, is not necessarily indicative of a disease process; therefore, answer 2 is correct.

Questions

Q25

The nurse is aware that in order to prevent the transmission of AIDS and other blood-borne pathogens in the healthcare setting she must do all of the following EXCEPT:

1) recap all needles and syringes
2) wash her hands before and after patient contact
3) consider all bodily fluids to be contaminated
4) don protective clothing and gloves during procedures

*Your Own Answer*_____

Q26

A 35-year-old woman is admitted to the medical unit of the hospital with the following symptoms: chronic fatigue, weight loss, diarrhea, night sweats, swollen inguinal lymph nodes, fever for the past month, and red and purple lesions on her legs and abdomen. The nurse takes appropriate action by:

1) wearing a mask, gloves, gown, and goggles during all patient contact
2) rooming this patient with a cancer patient receiving chemotherapy
3) placing labels on the chart and a sign outside the room that indicate the client's illness
4) wearing a mask, gown, and gloves only during contact involving bodily fluids

*Your Own Answer*_____

Correct Answers

A25

Answers 2, 3, and 4 are all appropriate behaviors for the prevention of transmission of AIDS and other blood-borne infectious diseases. Recapping needles and syringes is dangerous; they should be carefully placed, uncapped, in the nearest sharps container. Therefore, answer 1 is the correct choice.

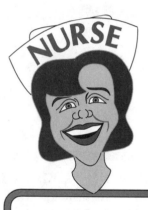

A26

This patient has many of the presenting signs and symptoms of AIDS. Answer 1 is therefore not the best choice, as it reflects the nurse's misunderstanding of the transmission modes for the disease and may make the patient feel stigmatized and feared. Answer 2 is not the best choice; two immunocompromised clients should not be roomed together. The actions in answer 3 are unnecessary and may lead to a double-standard of care for patients with AIDS. Answer 4 is correct and reflects the nurse's understanding of appropriate precautions when caring for a client with AIDS.

Questions

Q27

An obese elderly client has type II diabetes mellitus. The nurse spends considerable time teaching her about dietary management of the disease. The nurse knows that the teaching has been effective if the client states:

1) "I should lose weight as fast as I can in the first few months."
2) "I should eat a diet low in polyunsaturated fats."
3) "I will never be able to eat cake or ice cream again."
4) "I should eat more starches and fibers and less cake and ice cream."

*Your Own Answer*_____

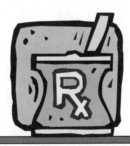

ACid   AlK
— 7.35.7.45
CO2 35 - 45

CO3 22-26

Q28

Respiratory <u>acidosis</u>, retention of excess carbon monoxide in the blood, is characterized by the following laboratory findings:

1) a pH < 7.35 and a PaC02 > 45 mmHg
2) a pH < 7.35 and an HC03- < 22 mEq/liter
3) a pH >7.42 and an HC03- < 22 mEq/liter
4) a pH >7.42 and a PaC02 < 35 mmHg

*Your Own Answer*_____

Correct Answers

A27

Answer 1 is incorrect; in the noninsulin-dependent diabetic, weight loss should occur gradually through dietary changes and exercise. Answer 2 is not a good choice; the diabetic should replace saturated (animal) fats with polyunsaturated (vegetable) fats. Answer 3 is a poor choice; the diabetic should limit the intake of refined sugars, but does not have to eliminate them altogether. Therefore, answer 4 is correct, demonstrating the correct emphasis on what is allowed, rather than what is forbidden.

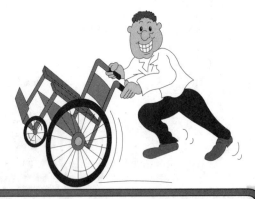

A28

Answer 1 is correct; these are the findings of uncompensated respiratory acidosis. Answer 2 shows the findings in uncompensated metabolic acidosis, answer 3 shows uncompensated metabolic alkalosis, and answer 4 lists findings for uncompensated respiratory alkalosis; therefore, these are all incorrect.

Questions

Q29

A hospitalized patient is vomiting and restless, has diarrhea, has a respiration rate of 8 to 10 per minute, and shows arrhythmias on the EKG monitor. The nurse is aware that these symptoms may be indicative of the acid-base imbalance:

1) metabolic acidosis
2) metabolic alkalosis
3) respiratory acidosis
4) respiratory alkalosis

*Your Own Answer*_____

Q30

Results for the arterial blood gas labs came back for a hospitalized client. The diagnosis is an acid-base disorder called respiratory alkalosis. The signs and symptoms that initially alerted the nurse to this client's condition were:

1) confusion, restlessness, and slow respirations
2) confusion, restlessness, and Kussmaul respirations
3) confusion, tingling of extremities, and deep, rapid respirations
4) confusion, tingling of extremities, and rapid, shallow respirations

*Your Own Answer*_____

Correct Answers

A29

Answer 2 is correct; these are the presumptive symptoms of metabolic alkalosis, which would be confirmed on arterial blood gas sampling. Answers 1, 3, and 4, therefore, are incorrect.

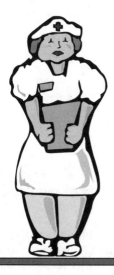

A30

Answer 3 correctly lists the classic signs and symptoms of respiratory alkalosis, in which there is an increased level of blood pH and a decrease in the $PaCO_2$ blood level. Answers 1, 2, and 4 present a mixture of symptoms of the other acid-base disorders—respiratory acidosis, metabolic acidosis, and metabolic alkalosis—and are therefore incorrect.

Questions

Q31

The nurse knows that her client understands her teaching when he states that the arterial blood gas (ABG) lab test is being performed to determine:

1) the blood pressure in his arteries
2) the amount of gas in his intestines
3) how efficiently his heart is pumping
4) the efficiency of respiratory ventilation

*Your Own Answer*_____

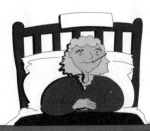

Q32

The following organs and glands are involved in the homeostatic process of controlling body fluid composition and volume:

1) lungs, heart, kidneys, adrenal glands, parathyroid glands, and pituitary gland
2) lungs, heart, kidneys, adrenal glands, pancreas, and pineal gland
3) lungs, heart, kidneys, adrenal glands, pancreas, and liver
4) lungs, heart, kidneys, small and large intestines, and liver

*Your Own Answer*_____

Correct Answers

A31

Alterations and disturbances in acid-base balance can be due to easily correctable problems such as hyperventilation or to such serious conditions as diabetic acidosis. The ABG is performed in order to evaluate ventilation, using blood pH, carbon dioxide, and carbonic acid level. Therefore, answer 4 is correct, and 1, 2, and 3 are all incorrect.

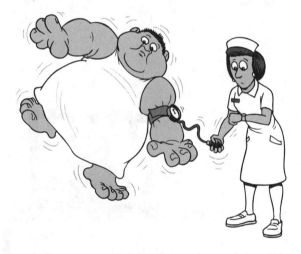

A32

Answer 1 is correct; these are the major glands and organs involved in blood circulation, removal of water through exhalation and excretion, and regulation of fluid and electrolyte balance. The other organs and glands mentioned in answers 2, 3, and 4 are not directly involved in the processes of body fluid homeostasis.

Questions

Q33

The process of inflammation involves all of the following EXCEPT:

1) heat and induration
2) tingling and itching
3) pain or tenderness
4) redness and edema

*Your Own Answer*_____

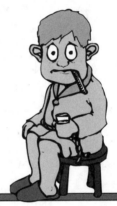

Q34

Atropine overdose is indicated by which of the following classic symptoms?

1) Confusion, flushed face, decreased body temperature, and increased secretions
2) Confusion, flushed face, increased body temperature, and increased thirst
3) Irritability, increased body temperature, increased secretions, and ashen color
4) Irritability, decreased body temperature, increased thirst, and ashen color

*Your Own Answer*_____

Correct Answers

A33

Answer 2 is the correct choice; inflammation involves all of the above except tingling and itching. Answers 1, 3, and 4 are therefore incorrect.

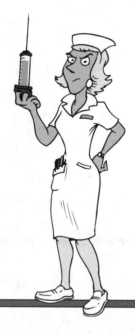

A34

Answer 2 is correct, listing the classic symptoms of atropine toxicity: "mad as a hatter, red as a beet, hot as a hare, and dry as a bone." Irritability, increased secretions, and ashen color do not characterize atropine overdose; therefore, answers 1, 3, and 4 are incorrect.

Questions

A client with acute liver failure has a decreased level of serum albumin. The nurse is aware that the most important interventions for this client include all of the following EXCEPT:

1) assess the client for signs and symptoms of dehydration
2) check the client for peripheral edema and ascites
3) offer high-protein foods and encourage intake of 50 g per day
4) assess for pitted edema and maintain skin integrity

*Your Own Answer*_____

An appropriate nursing diagnosis for an alcoholic client might be:

1) shame and guilt related to past and present problems with alcohol
2) acute memory loss and difficulty concentrating related to alcohol consumption
3) major depression related to feelings of worthlessness and hopelessness
4) altered nutrition: less than body requirement related to poor nutrition

*Your Own Answer*_____

Correct Answers

A35

Albumin, synthesized in the liver, increases osmotic pressure in the vessels, helping to maintain vessel fluid volume. With acute liver failure also usually comes decreased serum albumin, causing fluid to extravasate from the vessels to the tissues, resulting in edema. The interventions in answers 2, 3, and 4 are all important to the patient with hepatic failure. Dehydration, on the other hand, would not be an expected result of decreased albumin; therefore, answer 1 is correct.

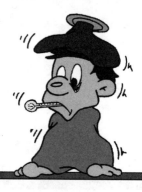

A36

Answer 1 is incorrect; shame and guilt are feelings, not a diagnosis. Answer 2 is also incorrect; these are symptoms, not a diagnosis. Answer 3 is a psychiatric diagnosis, not a nursing diagnosis, and is therefore incorrect. Therefore, answer 4 is the best choice; alcoholics generally develop nutritional deficiencies and may begin to lose weight as the craving for and consumption of alcohol replaces nutritious foods and beverages and meals occur in a haphazard and unpredictable manner.

Questions

Q37

The nurse knows that the client with Addison's disease needs to be assessed for the all of the following EXCEPT:

1) dehydration
2) overhydration
3) vital signs
4) GI discomfort

*Your Own Answer*_____

Q38

The nurse is acting in a responsible fashion in the administration of medication when she/he does all of the following EXCEPT:

1) evaluates the client's condition and compatibility with the medication
2) wears gloves and swabs the injection site with alcohol prior to injecting
3) administers the medication the client has been storing at the bedside
4) reviews the side effects and safety precautions of the medication

*Your Own Answer*_____

Correct Answers

A37

Addison's disease, caused by a deficiency of cortical hormones produced in the adrenal glands, can progress to the acute crisis stage characterized by acute hypotension (answer 3); nausea, diarrhea, and abdominal pain (answer 4); and chronic dehydration (answer 1). The nurse would not expect to see signs of overhydration; therefore, answer 2 is correct.

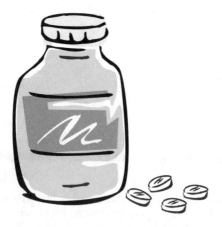

A38

Answer 3 is correct; medication should never be stored by the client's bedside, even if the client is to self-administer the medication. Answers 1, 2, and 4 indicate the nurse's understanding of the responsibilities in administering medications.

Questions

The nurse is aware that in order to evaluate the postoperative client for the respiratory complication of atelectasis, he/she should assess for:

1) bradycardia, rapid and shallow respirations, dry cough, and fever
2) tachycardia, rapid and shallow respirations, productive cough, and fever
3) tachycardia, asymmetrical chest movements, and decreased breath sound
4) bradycardia, asymmetrical chest movements, dry cough, and fever

*Your Own Answer*_____

Hypovolemic shock, a serious postoperative complication requiring rapid response by the nurse and/or physician, is indicated by:

1) increased urine output, increased blood pressure, cool clammy skin, and agitation
2) decreased urine output, decreased blood pressure, cool clammy skin, and agitation
3) increased urine output, decreased blood pressure, warm dry skin, and lethargy
4) decreased urine output, increased blood pressure, warm dry skin, and lethargy

*Your Own Answer*_____

Correct Answers

A39

Atelectasis ("collapsed" lung) is indicated by tachycardia, asymmetrical chest movements, and decreased breath sounds, as well as restlessness and dyspnea; therefore answer 3 is correct. Answer 2, incorrect, lists some of the symptoms of postoperative pneumonia. Bradycardia would not occur in the client having respiratory complications; therefore answers 1 and 4 are incorrect.

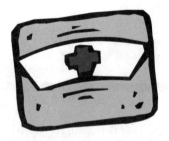

A40

Only answer 2 correctly lists some of the telltale symptoms of the client in hypovolemic shock, often due to postoperative hemorrhage. Therefore answers 1, 3, and 4 are incorrect.

Questions

Q41

The nurse recognizes the early signs of septic shock—fever, chills, dry flushed skin, altered mental status, increased pulse and respiration, decreased or normal blood pressure—in a client recently returned to the floor from surgery. The top priority interventions would be to:

1) give the regular medications and monitor vital signs and level of consciousness
2) alert the physician and give intravenous fluids to restore blood volume
3) administer oxygen and monitor vital signs and level of consciousness
4) help the client to ambulate, give oral fluids, and encourage frequent urination

*Your Own Answer*_____

Q42

The nurse is aware that complications of the GI tract can occur in the postoperative client. The most important assessments for early detection of paralytic ileus would be all of the following EXCEPT:

1) assess for abdominal distention by monitoring abdominal girth
2) auscultate for bowel sounds in all four quadrants
3) encourage ambulation and allow the client nothing by mouth
4) monitor flatus and the passage of stool

*Your Own Answer*_____

Correct Answers

A41

Septic shock, a possible postoperative complication due to a break in asepsis during surgery, occurs when bacteria enter the bloodstream and decrease vascular resistance, resulting in extreme hypotension. Answer 2 correctly indicates the priority nursing interventions for early-stage septic shock. Vital signs and LOC would be monitored often, once the physician had been notified and the patient rehydrated. Oxygen would most likely not be administered at the first signs of septic shock, the client would not be asked to ambulate or take oral fluids, nor would frequent urination be encouraged; therefore answers 1, 3, and 4 are not the best choices.

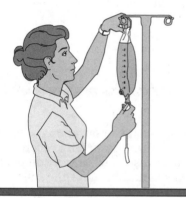

A42

Answers 1, 2, and 4 are all appropriate assessments for postoperative paralytic ileus. Answer 3 is the correct choice, as it is not an assessment but an intervention for the postoperative client with GI complications.

Questions

Q43

During assessment of the surgical client 36 hours postoperatively, the nurse notices that she has bowel sounds in only one quadrant, has passed no stool or flatus, is vomiting, and has a distended and tender abdomen. The nurse is aware that the appropriate interventions for this client would include:

1) observation for another 24 hours and assessment again for bowel sounds
2) forcing of fluids orally and through IV and immediate catheterization
3) contacting the physician immediately; this constitutes a serious emergency
4) nothing by mouth until bowel sounds return and encouragement of ambulation

*Your Own Answer*_____

Q44

Pulmonary embolism, a serious postoperative complication, should be suspected with the appearance of which of the following signs and symptoms?

1) chest pain, dyspnea, bradycardia, hypertension, cyanosis, and diaphoresis
2) chest pain, dyspnea, tachycardia, hypertension, cyanosis, and diaphoresis
3) chest pain, dyspnea, tachycardia, hypotension, cyanosis, and diaphoresis
4) chest pain, hyperventialtion, tachycardia, hypertension, cyanosis, and diaphoresis

*Your Own Answer*_____

Correct Answers

A43

This client is most likely suffering from postoperative paralytic ileus, a not uncommon complication stemming from the interruption of autonomic innervation of the GI tract. Answer 1 is therefore incorrect and indicates the nurse's lack of understanding of the importance of timely intervention to relieve the client's discomfort and prevent more serious GI complications. Answer 2, also incorrect, lists inappropriate interventions for paralytic ileus. Answer 3 is incorrect, as this situation does not yet constitute an emergency. The physician would be notified if the condition does not resolve within 24 to 48 more hours, at which time the physician might order a NG tube for feeding. Answer 4 is correct; these are the most appropriate interventions the nurse can make at this point to encourage the return of GI function.

A44

The correct signs and symptoms alerting the nurse to a pulmonary embolism, a blood clot usually originating in a leg vein that has lodged in the lung, are listed in answer 3. Answers 1, 2, and 4 are therefore incorrect.

Questions

Q45

Providing comfort for the postoperative client is an important nursing care goal. To accomplish this goal, the nurse most often should prioritize which intervention?

1) positioning of the client
2) administration of pain medication
3) bathing the client
4) feeding the client

*Your Own Answer*_____

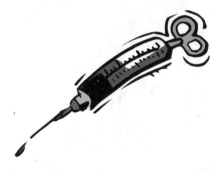

Q46

The most important immediate postoperative care goals include all of the following EXCEPT:

1) maintenance of respiratory function
2) maintenance of cardiovascular function
3) maintenance of fluid and electrolyte balance
4) maintenance of hygiene

*Your Own Answer*_____

Correct Answers

A45

Whenever possible, the nurse should provide comfort to the postoperative client through means other than pain medication. Therefore, answer 1 is the best choice. The other interventions, answers 2, 3, and 4, are all important interventions postoperatively, but are not the first priority in providing comfort.

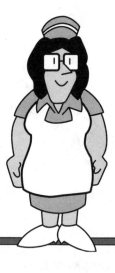

A46

The maintenance of the postoperative client's hygiene is not among the top priority nursing interventions in the immediate postsurgical period, although it is a meaningful measure toward the client's comfort; therefore, answer 4 is the correct choice. Answers 1, 2, and 3 all are included among the most important nursing interventions immediately postoperative.

Questions

Fluid and electrolyte balance is an important aspect of the postsurgical client's nursing care. This can be maintained through which of the following interventions?

I.   assessment of GI drainage
II. use of appropriate IV fluid and rate
III. assessment of oral temperature q 4 h
IV. assessment of renal function lab values

1) I, II, and III
2) II, III, and IV
3) I, II, and IV
4) all of the above

*Your Own Answer*_____

Appropriate interventions for the maintenance of respiratory function in the postoperative client would include all of the following EXCEPT:

1) deep breathing and coughing
2) use of an incentive spirometer
3) chest physiotherapy
4) elevation of the feet 45 degrees

*Your Own Answer*_____

Correct Answers

A47

Assessment of the client's temperature will not give the most relevant information regarding postoperative fluid and electrolyte balance. However, all three other interventions are important in accomplishing this goal. Therefore, answer 3 is correct, and answers 1, 2, and 4 are not.

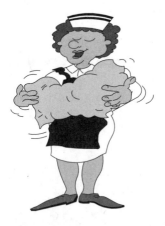

A48

All three interventions in answers 1, 2, and 3 are important to the maintenance of respiratory function, especially in a bedridden postoperative client. Therefore, answer 4 is the correct choice: raising the foot of the bed to elevate the feet 45 degrees is not an appropriate intervention; however, raising the *head* of the bed might be appropriate to increase drainage of respiratory secretions.

Questions

Ms. H. has been in the recovery room for the past few hours. The nurse knows that she will not be returned to the medical-surgical floor until all of the following are present:

1) vital signs are stable, client is awake, dressings are intact, and airway is patent
2) vital signs are stable, client is awake, bowel sounds are heard in all four quadrants
3) vital signs are stable, client is awake, client can deep breathe and cough
4) vital signs are stable, client is awake, dressings are intact, client can take oral fluids

*Your Own Answer*_____

The nurse knows that the client understands the postoperative teaching when he states:

1) "There must be something very wrong; I haven't yet urinated and I had surgery 4 hours ago."
2) "If everything goes well, I can expect to urinate spontaneously sometime after 12 hours postsurgery."
3) "I had my surgery 15 hours ago and still haven't urinated, but you said it can take up to 24 hours."
4) "I will expect the urinary catheter to be removed and to urinate on my own beginning right after surgery."

*Your Own Answer*_____

Correct Answers

A49

The correct answer is 1: these are the four most basic requirements for release from the recovery room. Bowel sounds would not be expected to be audible immediately postsurgery, as the client has been NPO for many hours at this point; therefore, answer 2 is incorrect. Deep breathing and coughing, in answer 3, would also not be expected prior to release from the recovery room. Neither would the client be expected to take oral fluids, in answer 4, until the return of normal GI function postoperatively.

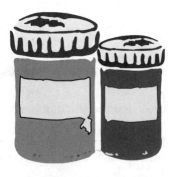

A50

Answer 2 is correct; barring any postoperative complications involving urinary retention, the nurse teaches the client that spontaneous voiding cannot be expected within the first 12 hours. Therefore, answers 1, 3, and 4 are incorrect.

Questions

Q51

Sixteen hours after undergoing abdominal surgery, Mr. F. is complaining of pain just above the level of the symphysis pubis, and he is restless and anxious. The nurse also notes diaphoresis, increased blood pressure from 120/80 preoperatively to 160/95, and a normal temperature and pulse. The nurse suspects which postoperative complication:

1) surgical wound infection
2) paralytic ileus
3) pulmonary embolism
4) urinary retention

*Your Own Answer*_____

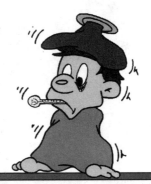

Q52

The priority nursing goals of proper wound care include all of the following EXCEPT:

1) prevention of infection
2) promotion of comfort
3) measurement of drainage
4) promotion of dehiscence

*Your Own Answer*_____

Correct Answers

A51

Mr F. has the signs and symptoms of urinary retention, a normal finding within the first 12 hours postoperatively which is usually reversible and transient; therefore, answer 4 is correct. With wound infection, answer 1, one would expect an increased pulse rate and temperature. Paralytic ileus, answer 2, would be indicated by abdominal distention and possibly nausea and vomiting. Pulmonary embolism, answer 3, would involve chest pain and a decrease in blood pressure.

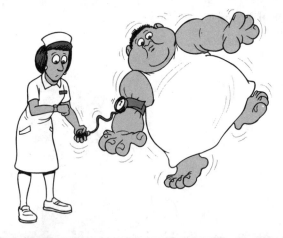

A52

Answer 4 is the correct choice; dehiscence, the process by which the layers of a surgical wound separate—often leading to evisceration—is to be avoided. The three other methods of wound care in answers 1, 2, and 3 are appropriate priority postsurgical measures.

Questions

Ms. R. returned from shoulder surgery three days ago. The nurse, in changing her dressing, notes her complaint of pain and tenderness at the incision site, as well as edema. Ms. R.'s lab results report an increased white blood cell count. From the last nursing shift, the chart indicates a temperature of 101 degrees and a pulse rate of 96. The nurse's priority interventions should include which of the following:

1) administer antibiotics as ordered, perform a dipstick urinalysis, and keep the wound dressing intact for the next 24 hours
2) administer antibiotics as ordered, obtain a wound culture and sensitivity test, and irrigate the wound
3) administer the usual medications, encourage ambulation, and keep the wound dressing intact for the next 12 hours
4) no special measures need to be taken; this is the expected postsurgical response

*Your Own Answer*_____

The nurse ascertains that the client is prepared for surgery when all of the following have been done preoperatively EXCEPT:

1) jewelry and dentures removed from the client
2) identification bands removed from the client
3) skin preparation at the incision site
4) NPO status has been confirmed

*Your Own Answer*_____

Correct Answers

A53

The correct answer is 2; this client has the signs and symptoms of a surgical wound infection. Administration of antibiotics and frequent irrigation of the wound with the appropriate solution are essential to avoiding further complications, such as dehiscence and evisceration. Ambulation, in answer 3, would not be encouraged in a patient with a wound infection. Dipstick urinalysis, in answer 1, is not immediately relevant to wound infection assessment or treatment. Answer 4, not a good response, reflects the nurse's lack of understanding of the necessity of attention to postsurgical wound infection.

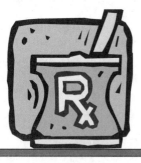

A54

Answer 2 is the correct choice; ID bands must remain on the surgical client at all times, as the client will be transported from the unit to the receiving area, OR, and recovery room by varied personnel. The ID band will be matched to the one attached to the client's chart at all stages of the surgical process. The procedures enumerated in answers 1, 3, and 4 are part of the preop preparation and are therefore not the correct choices.

Questions

Q55

Medical asepsis, accomplished through thorough and routine handwashing and by wearing (nonsterile) clean gloves, is important in the administration of which of the following:

I. dirty linen removal
II. tube feedings
III. administration of medications
IV. client hygiene

1) I, II, and III
2) II, III, and IV
3) I, II, and IV
4) all of the above

*Your Own Answer*_____

Q56

"Sterile technique," also known as surgical asepsis, is used in which of the following procedures:

1) surgery, catheterizations, vaginal delivery of a baby, and dressing changes
2) surgery, catheterizations, testing of urine by dipstick analysis, and dressing changes
3) surgery, catheter removals, vaginal delivery of a baby, and dressing changes
4) surgery, catheter removals, phlebotomy, and dressing changes

*Your Own Answer*_____

Correct Answers

A55

Answer 2 is correct. Handwashing is not necessary for the removel of dirty linens. However, it is recommended that nonsterile gloves be worn during the removal of dirty linens for the protection of the nurse's hands and prevention of infection spread. Medical asepsis should be observed while making the client's bed with fresh linens. Therefore, answers 1, 3, and 4 are not the best choices.

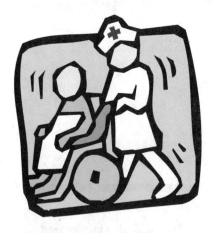

A56

The correct choice is answer 1. Catheter removal, dipstick urinalysis, and phlebotomy do not require surgical asepsis, although medical asepsis is important in these procedures. Therefore, answers 2, 3, and 4 are incorrect.

Questions

Q57

Steps in the nursing process include which of the following:

1) assessment, communication, planning, implementation, and evaluation
2) diagnosis, planning, organizing, implementation, and analysis
3) assessment, diagnosis, planning, implementation, and evaluation
4) fact gathering, diagnosis, communication, planning, and evaluation

*Your Own Answer*_____

Q58

The nurse is certain that the client teaching was effective regarding the proper acid ash diet for urinary tract infection treatment and prevention when the client states:

1) "I will add peaches, pears, papayas, and strawberries to my usual diet."
2) "I will add nuts, berries, watermelon, and mushrooms to my usual diet."
3) "I will eat more yellow and leafy green vegetables in my daily diet."
4) "I will add prunes, plums, and unsweetened cranberry juice to my diet."

*Your Own Answer*_____

Correct Answers

A57

Answer 3 correctly lists the commonly agreed-upon steps in the nursing process. Therefore, answers 1, 2, and 4 are incorrect.

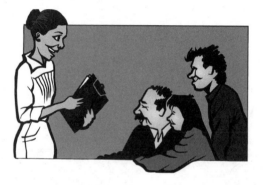

A58

The client reflects her understanding of the foods that are acidic and contain ash in answer 4, which is correct. These foods help create and/or maintain an acidic environment in the urinary tract, "unfriendly" to most bacteria that would otherwise colonize there. Therefore, answers 1, 2, and 3 are incorrect.

Questions

Q59

Discharge planning for the surgical client should begin:

1) immediately postsurgery, in the recovery room if possible
2) during first contact with the client, preferably preoperatively
3) two to three days postsurgically so as not to upset the client
4) immediately preoperatively, perhaps on the way to the OR

*Your Own Answer*_____

Q60

After a central venous (CV) line has been surgically inserted, the nurse knows that the line must be maintained by:

1) flushing the catheter on a regular basis to keep it patent and changing the injection cap from time to time
2) replacing the catheter tubing every 24 to 48 hours and changing the dressing at least once a week or when soiled
3) flushing all lumens of a multilumen catheter with either 0. 9% sodium chloride or heparinized saline
4) performing all of the above

*Your Own Answer*_____

Correct Answers

A59

Answer 2 is correct and reflects the nurse's understanding of the importance of discharge planning. Planning can begin with the initial client assessment and history-taking, and should include consideration of psychosocial, economic, physical, and nutritional factors. Answers 1 and 4 are incorrect; they reflect unreasonable expectations and would be upsetting to the client. Answer 3 is also not a good choice; discharge planning takes time, including making arrangements for transport to and care at home; medication administration at home; and many types of client and family/caregiver teaching.

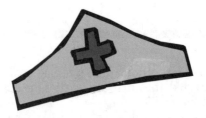

A60

Answer 4 is correct; all of the above procedures are important to the maintenance of a CV line. Answers 1, 2, and 3 by themselves are not the best choices.

Questions

Q61

The client with a disposable external colostomy pouch demonstrates understanding of the post-operative teaching when he states:

1) "I must change the pouch if a leak develops and should empty it when it's half full."
2) "I should wait until the pouch is full to empty it to avoid irritating the ostomy site."
3) "I can reuse the pouch for up to two weeks as long as I empty it frequently enough."
4) both answers 1 and 3

*Your Own Answer*_____

Q62

Which of the following are risk factors for the development of renal calculi:

I.   urinary stasis
II. immobility
Ill. being female and > 40 years old
IV. hypercalcemia

1) I, II, and Ill
2) II, Ill, and IV
3) I, II, and IV
4) all of the above

*Your Own Answer*_____

Correct Answers

A61

Answer 1 is the best choice. The pouch should be emptied when it is about one-third to half full; waiting until it is completely full can result in leaking or oozing of fecal matter around the ostomy site. Most disposable systems can be used for 2 to 7 days at most, not two weeks. The system should be changed if a leak develops. Therefore, answers 2, 3, and 4 are not the best choices.

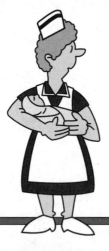

A62

"Urolithiasis" refers to stones formed anywhere within the urinary system by the deposit of crystalized substances excreted in the urine, such as calcium oxalate and uric acid. Urinary stasis, prolonged immobility due to illness, and hypercalcemia are all conditions favoring the formation of kidney stones. Being male, not female, and over 40 years of age are also risk factors. Therefore, answer 3 is the best choice, and answers 1, 2, and 4 are incorrect.

Questions

A 52-year-old male enters the emergency room complaining of blood in his urine and severe pain in his lower back that radiates down into his flank area and which comes and goes in waves. He has been nauseous and vomiting for the past two days, and has had occasional diarrhea as well. The ER nurse suspects this client is suffering from:

1) a peptic ulcer, and will prepare the client for a lower GI series
2) renal calculi, and will prepare the client for intravenous urography
3) chronic renal failure, and will draw blood for BUN and serum creatinine levels
4) pyelonephritis, and will obtain a urine culture and sensitivity test

*Your Own Answer*_____

The prevention of recurrent urinary tract infections is one of the goals of the nurse in the community clinic setting. The nurse knows that the young women clients understand the information she has presented when they state all of the following EXCEPT:

1) "It is better to take showers than to take baths."
2) "We should remember to urinate after intercourse."
3) "After a BM, wiping back to front is the best way."
4) "We should try to avoid using perfumed toilet paper."

*Your Own Answer*_____

Correct Answers

A63

The client with a peptic ulcer would most likely present with a dull, gnawing pain, and would not have hematuria, though vomiting is not unusual; furthermore, an *upper, not a lower,* GI series would be ordered for this client. Therefore, answer 1 is incorrect. Chronic renal failure, in its earliest stage, might be asymptomatic, although as it progresses weakness and fatigue as well as polyuria are the main presenting symptoms. Therefore, answer 3 is incorrect. Pyelonephritis is usually accompanied by chills and fever, and often dysuria and frequency. Therefore, answer 4 is not the best choice. The best answer is 2; these are the classic symptoms of kidney "stones."

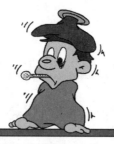

A64

Answers 1, 2, and 4 all indicate the clients' understanding of the nurse's recommendations for the prevention of UTIs. Answer 3 is the correct choice, as this demonstrates faulty understanding; it is always best to wipe from front to back both after a bowel movement and after urination to avoid the mechanical transfer of bacteria across the perineum to the urethral opening (as well as to the vagina).

Questions

Q65

Cystitis, or infection of the bladder, is seen most frequently among young women. Which of the following symptoms would alert the nurse to the possibility of this UTI?

1) burning upon urination
2) urinary frequency and urgency
3) hematuria and fever
4) all of the above

*Your Own Answer*_____

Q66

The immediate postmastectomy client can be expected to have concerns reflecting her altered body image. The nurse's best response to the client's statement, "I am afraid my husband won't find me attractive any more," would be:

1) "There will be plenty of time to talk about that later on. Right now you have to focus on your recovery from the surgery."
2) "Many men do find it difficult to adjust to their wives' new physical shape. Your husband probably isn't any different."
3) "You are expressing a common fear many women have after this surgery. I'd like to hear more about your feelings."
4) "After the reconstruction surgery you will look as good as new. Your husband will hardly know the difference."

*Your Own Answer*_____

Correct Answers

A65

Answers 1, 2, and 3 are all correct in listing the most common symptoms of cystitis, along with suprapubic pain, and nausea and vomiting; therefore answer 4 is the best choice.

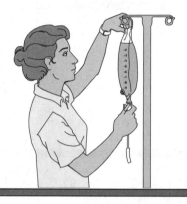

A66

In answer 1, the nurse shows a lack of awareness for the "healing potential" in focusing on the client's psychological concerns as they naturally arise; therefore, this is not a good choice. Answer 2 is very unsupportive and may reflect the nurse's own uncomfortableness with sexuality and intimacy; this is therefore not the best answer. In answer 4, also not a good choice, the nurse assumes that the client will choose reconstructive surgery and denies the seriousness of this client's concerns. Only answer 3 reflects an understanding of this client's need to talk, as well as the nurse's therapeutic "offer of the self." Answer 3 is therefore the best choice.

Questions

Q67

The nurse's top priority goals for the postmastectomy client include all of the following EXCEPT:

1) elevate the arm of the affected side, with distal joint higher than proximal joint
2) assess frequently for the signs and symptoms of edema and infection
3) monitor vital signs and perform venipuncture on the nonaffected side
4) begin arm exercises no sooner than the first 72 hours postsurgery

*Your Own Answer*_____

Q68

In order to ascertain that a nasogastric tube has been properly inserted, the nurse:

1) asks the client if he or she can feel the tube wending its way down the esophagus to the stomach
2) attaches a 10-cc syringe to the tube and gently injects air while auscultating the abdomen for a "whoosh"
3) attaches the feeding tube to the nutritional solution and starts the drip to see if it backs up
4) attaches a 10-cc syringe to the tube and quickly injects NS while auscultating the abdomen for a "swish"

*Your Own Answer*_____

Correct Answers

A67

Answers 1, 2, and 3 all indicate the correct approach to postsurgical care of the client with a mastectomy. Arm exercises should begin within the first 24 hours postsurgery in order to maintain the full range of motion of the affected-side shoulder joint. Therefore, answer 4 is the best choice.

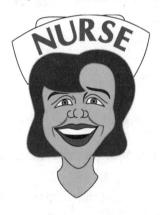

A68

Only the procedure in answer 2, the best choice, will safely tell the nurse that the NG tube has successfully reached its destination of the stomach. An x-ray can also confirm this. Therefore, answers 1, 3, and 4 are incorrect.

Questions

Q69

A nasogastric feeding tube should be removed:
1) as slowly as possible, after distracting the client
2) as quickly as possible, after distracting the client
3) as slowly as possible, after informing the client
4) quickly and gently, after informing the client

*Your Own Answer*_____

Q70

In teaching a client's family member how to care for the feeding tube at home, the nurse explains which of the following actions:

I. Assess tube placement by aspirating gastric contents using a syringe
II. Flush the feeding tube q 8 hrs, with 40-60 cc NS to maintain patency
III. Retape the tube at least daily and inspect skin for redness and breakdown
IV. Assist with oral hygiene—tooth and gum brushing—at least twice a day

1) I, II, and III
2) II, III, and IV
3) I, II, and IV
4) all of the above

*Your Own Answer*_____

Correct Answers

Answer 4 is the best choice. After explaining the procedure to the client, the nurse will quickly though gently withdraw the tube from the stomach, esophagus, and nose. Therefore, answers 1, 2, and 3 are not the best choices.

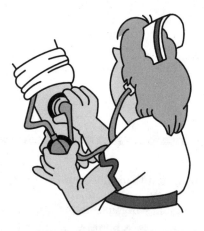

Answer 2 is the best choice. Each of these three procedures would be easily performed by a family member. It would not, however, be appropriate to teach a family member to perform the assessment of tube placement by gastric-content aspiration. This would be more appropriately done by a visiting or home-care nurse. Answers 1, 3, and 4 are therefore not the best choices.

Questions

A woman in her second trimester of pregnancy is used to sleeping on her back. She asks the nurse if this is acceptable throughout the rest of the prenatal period. The nurse's best recommendation would be:

1) "Sleep in any comfortable position."
2) "On your back is preferable."
3) "Sleep with your feet and head elevated 30-45 degrees."
4) "Sleep on either your left or right side."

*Your Own Answer*_____

Alpha fetoprotein (AFP) serum screening is a laboratory test done during pregnancy

1) between 16 and 20 weeks to detect open neural tube defect
2) between 16 and 20 weeks to detect hyperbilirubinemia
3) between 8 and 12 weeks to detect multiple gestations
4) between 8 and 12 weeks to detect phenylketonuria

*Your Own Answer*_____

Correct Answers

A71

All positions other than left or right side-lying are unsafe for prolonged periods of time, and can cause vena-cava syndrome. Side-lying promotes uterine perfusion and fetoplacental oxygenation. Therefore, answer 4 is the nurse's best recommendation and answers 1, 2, and 3 would not be good choices.

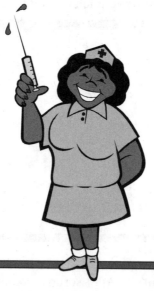

A72

Answer 1 is correct; amniocentesis and ultrasound may also be used to detect neural tube defect in the fetus. Hyperbilirubinemia and phenylketonuria, answers 2 and 4, are detected through other blood work in the neonate, not the fetus; therefore these answers are incorrect. Multiple gestations, answer 3, could be detected through AFP, but not as early as 8 to 12 weeks; this answer is therefore incorrect.

Questions

A 23-year old woman presents at the GYN clinic for her annual pelvic exam. While taking her medical history, the nurse learns that the client is sexually active with several different partners, and reports the following symptoms at this visit: dysuria; polyuria; lower abdominal pain; dyspareunia; and a malodorous, frothy, yellow-green vaginal discharge. The nurse is aware that the client may have contracted:

1) candidiasis
2) trichomoniasis
3) human papillomavirus (HPV)
4) chlamydia

*Your Own Answer*_____

Twelve hours after birth, a newborn appears jaundiced. A serum bilirubin level is obtained and is 14 mg/dl. The nurse's plan of care for the baby will be based on her awareness that:

1) immediate intervention is required for severe hyperbilirubinemia
2) these are normal manifestations of physiologic jaundice
3) this occurs in breastfed babies receiving only colostrum during the first days
4) these are signs of breast-milk jaundice; this newborn is well

*Your Own Answer*_____

Correct Answers

A73

Symptoms of all four infections may include dysuria and dyspareunia. However, only trichomoniasis presents with a complaint of polyuria and a malodorous, frothy, yellow-green vaginal discharge; therefore answer 2 is correct. In candidiasis, the vaginal discharge is thick, white, and cheeselike in texture; therefore, 1 is not the correct answer. HPV usually causes dry, wartlike growths on the vulva, vagina, cervix, and rectum, and no vaginal discharge; therefore, 3 is not correct. Answer 4 is incorrect because a purulent discharge and cervical bleeding may be present with chlamydia, or the woman may be asymptomatic and diagnosis is only made on Pap smear.

A74

Answer 1 is correct; severe hyperbilirubinemia, requiring immediate intervention to prevent brain damage, has its onset during the first 24 hours after birth and is diagnosed by a serum bilirubin level of >12.9 mg/dl in full-term infants. Answer 2 is incorrect, as physiologic jaundice doesn't appear until 24 hours after birth. Answer 3 is incorrect; jaundice that occurs in breastfed infants usually appears on day 2 or 3. Breast-milk jaundice, also called late-onset jaundice, begins 4 to 5 days after birth; therefore, answer 4 is incorrect.

Questions

Q75

The presumptive signs and symptoms of pregnancy correctly include which of the following:

1) positive urine pregnancy test, enlarged abdomen, and Braxton-Hicks contractions
2) positive urine pregnancy test, amenorrhea, fatigue, and softening of the cervix
3) increase in urination, amenorrhea, fatigue, breast enlargement, and quickening
4) increase in urination, amenorrhea, fatigue, enlarged abdomen, and fetal heartbeat

*Your Own Answer*_____

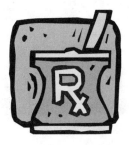

Q76

On examination of the prenatal client, the nurse is aware that she will assess for a bluish pigmentation of the vagina. This probable sign of pregnancy is also known as:

1) Hegar's sign
2) Chadwick's sign
3) Nightingale's sign
4) Goodell's sign

*Your Own Answer*_____

Correct Answers

A75

Only answer 3 correctly lists some of the presumptive signs and symptoms of pregnancy. A positive urine pregnancy teat, enlarged abdomen, Braxton-Hicks contractions, and a softening of the cervix (called Goodell's sign) are all probable signs of pregnancy. Presence of a fetal heartbeat is a positive sign of pregnancy. Therefore, answers 1, 2, and 4 are incorrect.

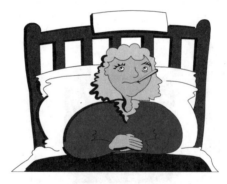

A76

Bluish pigmentation of the vagina in pregnancy is referred to as Chadwick's sign; therefore answer 2 is the correct choice. Hegar's sign refers to the softening of the uterus, felt on palpation. Goodell's sign is the softening of the cervical lip, apparent on the internal pelvic exam. There is no sign called Nightingale's sign. Therefore, answers 1, 3, and 4 are all incorrect.

Questions

Q77

In her prenatal teaching, the nurse informs the client that bloods will be drawn to check for antibodies (past exposure and present immunity) for the rubella virus. The nurse goes on to explain that if the client is antibody-negative, she will be given a rubella vaccination:

1) 6 weeks into her second trimester of pregnancy
2) 6 weeks into her third trimester of pregnancy
3) within 6 weeks of delivery of this baby
4) within 6 months of delivery of this baby

*Your Own Answer*_____

Q78

In order to determine the expected date of childbirth, the nurse uses Naegele's rule. This entails:

1) adding 3 months and 7 days to the date of the last menstrual period
2) subtracting 3 months and 7 days from the date of the last menstrual period
3) subtracting 3 months from the last menstrual period and then adding 7 days
4) adding 3 months to the last menstrual period and then subtracting 7 days

*Your Own Answer*_____

Correct Answers

A77

Rubella vaccination is recommended for women in the immediate postpartum period in order to prevent birth defects in future pregnancies. Therefore, answer 3 is the best choice. However, because the vaccine itself may be teratogenic, contraception should be used for at least 3 months after vaccination. The vaccine, therefore, would not be administered during pregnancy, and six months after childbirth might be too long to wait to administer the vaccine in women who continue to be sexually active. Therefore, answers 1, 2, and 4 are not the best choices.

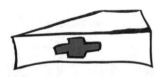

A78

Only answer 3 correctly indicates the method for calculating the estimated date of delivery according to Naegele's rule. Therefore, answers 1, 2, and 4 are all incorrect.

Questions

Q79

Which of the following signs of pregnancy will the nurse teach her prenatal clients are possible or to be expected in the next 6 to 7 months:

I.   increased need for oxygen and elevated diaphragm muscle
II. increased skin pigmentation, facial "mask," and linea nigra
Ill. increased motility of the GI tract, diarrhea, and vomiting
IV. increased heart rate, palpitations, and nosebleeds

1) I, II, and III
2) II, III, and IV
3) I, III, and IV
4) I, II, and IV

*Your Own Answer*_____

Q80

The first-time parents of a 2-day-old baby girl can be seen to be demonstrating positive adaptive behaviors when the postpartum nurse notes that:

1) they are both planning to attend a baby care class offered by the hospital nursing staff that afternoon
2) they are making plans to go away on a weeklong vacation next month while the grandparents watch the baby
3) they are handling the baby roughly, find changing the diapers "disgusting," and let the nurse bathe the baby
4) they allow the baby to cry for hours at a time because they are worried about raising a "spoiled" child

*Your Own Answer*_____

Correct Answers

Answer 4 is correct; these are all signs the prenatal client can be prepared to experience during the course of the pregnancy. *Decreased* GI tract motility and constipation, not diarrhea, would be expected. Therefore, answers 1, 2, and 3 are not good choices.

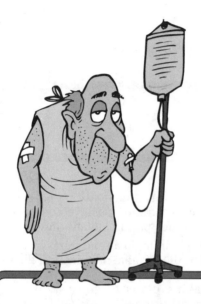

In answers 2, 3, and 4, the parents are responding inappropriately to the needs of the new baby and to their new responsibilities. New parents taking an active interest in the needs of the baby is indicative of a positive adaptive response to the "crisis" of new parenthood. Therefore, answer 1 is the best choice.

Questions

Q81

The nurse in the women's health clinic is performing an assessment on a 43-year-old woman, who reports difficulty sleeping, a feeling of warmth in her chest and face several times a day, vaginal dryness and painful intercourse, difficulty concentrating, decreased libido, and fatigue and irritability. The lab results in her chart show a normal CBC, an FSH of 40 IU/L, and an estrogen level of 18 pg/mL. The nurse suspects that this client is experiencing the signs and symptoms of:

1) an ectopic pregnancy
2) a vaginal infection
3) a urinary tract infection
4) menopause

*Your Own Answer*_____

Q82

The health clinic nurse teaches her 40- to 55-year-old female clients that most postmenopausal women are normally concerned about all of the following EXCEPT:

1) becoming pregnant
2) loss of sexual interest
3) difficulty falling asleep
4) mood swings and irritability

*Your Own Answer*_____

Correct Answers

A81

These are the positive signs and symptoms expected in the menopausal woman. Hot flashes and vaginal atrophy are a result of decreased levels of circulating estrogen, while the other symptoms may be a result of fluctuating levels of progesterone and other "female" hormones. Decreased libido may be a result of a decrease in circulating androgens. The labs indicate the classic low estrogen/increased FSH indicative of a diagnosis of menopause. Therefore, answer 4 is correct, and answers 1, 2, and 3 are not the best choices.

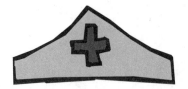

A82

"Postmenopausal" refers to women who have been at least a full year without a menstrual period and whose estrogen levels are not high enough to support the development of a mature follicle. Becoming pregnant, therefore, is not a usual concern of the woman at least a year past the onset of menopause. Therefore, answer 1 is correct. The three other symptoms are seen in up to 80 percent of postmenopausal women. Answers 2, 3, and 4 are not, therefore, the best choices.

Questions

Q83

The nurse teaches her prenatal clients that it is important to gain weight throughout their pregnancies. Which of the following average-weight-gain patterns is considered most healthy for a normal-weight mother during pregnancy:

1) 2 to 5 pounds per month in the first trimester and 1.5 to 2 pounds weekly thereafter
2) 2 to 5 pounds total in the first trimester and 0.66 to 1.1 pounds weekly thereafter
3) 0.5 to 1 pound total in the first trimester and 0.66 to 1.1 pounds weekly thereafter
4) 25 to 35 pounds within the first two trimesters and 1 to 2 pounds total in the third

Your Own Answer _____

Q84

Ellen is a 26-year-old in week 22 of her first pregnancy. She is at the clinic for a prenatal checkup and the nurse determines that appropriate nursing diagnoses include (1) altered nutrition: more than body requirement and (2) constipation. All of the following nursing interventions would be important for this client EXCEPT:

1) encourage Ellen to get regular exercise, such as swimming or brisk walking, throughout the rest of the pregnancy
2) identify the high-calorie foods in Ellen's current diet and plan daily menus of appealing, nutritious, low-calorie foods
3) remind Ellen that she should take better care of herself and her baby by eating a better diet and losing some weight
4) plan a diet with Ellen of high-fiber foods and fresh fruits and encourage her to drink 30 to 40 ml/kg of water each day

Your Own Answer _____

Correct Answers

A83

The correct answer is 2; the lower rate is for overweight women and the higher for underweight women. Poor weight gain and excessive weight gain during pregnancy are associated with various risks to both mother and baby. Answers 1, 3, and 4 therefore are incorrect.

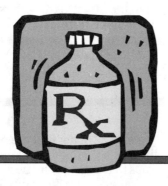

A84

Encouraging Ellen to get regular exercise and to replace high-calorie with low-calorie foods are two good ways of helping Ellen to slow down her weight gain throughout the remainder of her pregnancy. A diet of high-fiber foods and an increase in water intake will help soften stools and ease constipation. Therefore, the recommendations in answers 1, 2, and 4 are good interventions. The nurse's attitude in answer 3, the correct choice, is reprimanding and judgmental and therefore not of therapeutic benefit to this client. Furthermore, the client must not be encouraged to lose weight, but rather to gain more slowly for the rest of the pregnancy.

Questions

Q85

Appropriate iron intake—often involving supplementation to the regular diet—is very important during the course of pregnancy because:

1) the fetus makes its own iron during gestation and shares some with the mother; if intake is too low, not enough will replace fetal iron
2) the mother transfers about 300 mg of iron to the fetus during gestation; if iron intake is too low, it will cause anemia in the mother
3) the mother loses iron through urination, which becomes very frequent especially during the last trimester of pregnancy
4) iron is needed for the process of fetal calcification; most women don't get enough iron through diet to properly support this process

*Your Own Answer*_____

Q86

The nurse teaches her prenatal clients that the foods highest in protein, vital to the growth of the fetus, include:

1) green peppers, onions, avacado, beets, corn, and squash
2) oranges, grapefruit, lemons, grapes, melon, and kiwi
3) spinach, broccoli, potatoes, tomatoes, and string beans
4) milk, meat, cheese, eggs, kidney beans, and peanut butter

*Your Own Answer*_____

Correct Answers

A85

If enough iron is not available through diet to meet the needs of the mother, fetus, and placenta, reserves of fetal iron will not be disturbed. Babies are born with high hemoglobin levels and enough iron stored in the liver for 3 to 6 months. However, maternal red blood cell mass will be reduced and hemoglobin levels will decline more than usual during pregnancy, resulting in iron-deficiency anemia. This may leave the mother vulnerable in the event of a hemorrhage at the time of delivery. Therefore, answer 2 is correct, and answer 1 is incorrect. Iron is not lost through an increase in the frequency of urination; therefore, answer 3 is incorrect. The process of fetal calcification involves calcium, not iron; therefore answer 4 is also incorrect.

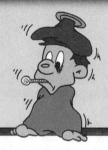

A86

Only answer 4 correctly lists the most common sources of dietary protein. Peanut butter should be eaten in small quantities, as it is high in fat and calories. All of the other foods listed in incorrect answers 1, 2, and 3 can be an important part of the pregnant woman's diet as a source of nutrients other than protein.

 Take Test-Readiness Quiz 1 on CD
(to review questions 1–86)

Questions

Blood

Q87

Placenta previa, a potentially serious maternal hemorrhagic complication of late pregnancy, can be identified by:

1) painless, bright red uterine bleeding in the third trimester
2) dark red vaginal bleeding with mild to severe pain
3) dark brown bleeding with nausea, vomiting, and fever
4) all of the above at various times throughout the pregnancy

*Your Own Answer*_____

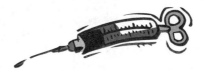

Q88

The major potential maternal hazard from pregnancy-induced hypertension (PIH) is:

1) nausea and vomiting
2) maternal infection
3) eclampsia (seizures)
4) low birth weight

*Your Own Answer*_____

Correct Answers

A87

Answer 1 correctly describes the most common presenting signs of placenta previa, the implantation of the placenta in a lower uterine segment, partially or completely covering the cervical os. Answer 2 is incorrect; these are the signs of abruptio placentae, the premature separation of the placenta from the uterus. Answer 3 is also incorrect; these signs are not related to any specific late pregnancy bleeding condition. Therefore, answer 4 is incorrect as well.

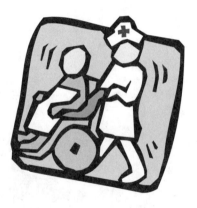

A88

If PIH goes untreated and progresses to preeclampsia, also left untreated, the result may be tonic/clonic convulsions, coma, and possibly death during pregnancy or shortly after birth. Answer 3 is therefore the correct answer. Answers 1, 2, and 4 are incorrect.

Questions

Q89

In order to control the convulsions or seizures that may result in the pregnant woman with severe preeclampsia, the nurse will:

1) administer calcium gluconate intravenously, as ordered by the physician
2) administer magnesium sulfate intravenously, as ordered by the physician
3) administer calcium citrate intramuscularly, as ordered by the physician
4) administer terbutaline intravenously, then orally, as ordered by the physician

*Your Own Answer*_____

Q90

A severely preeclamptic client is receiving magnesium sulfate in order to prevent convulsions. The nurse is aware that the signs and symptoms of magnesium sulfate toxicity include:

1) decrease in respirations; increase in blood pressure, pulse, and urinary output; sudden increase in fetal heart rate
2) increase in respirations, blood pressure, and pulse; decrease in urinary output; sudden increase in fetal heart rate
3) decrease in respirations, blood pressure, pulse, and urinary output; sudden drop in fetal heart rate
4) increase in respirations, blood pressure, pulse, and urinary output; sudden drop in fetal heart rate

*Your Own Answer*_____

Correct Answers

A89

Answer 2 is correct; magnesium sulfate is an anticonvulsant and smooth muscle relaxant used in the prevention of convulsions. Calcium gluconate is an antidote for magnesium sulfate, administered in the case of MgSO4 toxicity. Calcium citrate is a dietary supplement, usually taken by mouth and bought over the counter. Terbutaline is a smooth muscle relaxant, but used in cases of premature onset of labor. Therefore, answers 1, 3, and 4 are incorrect.

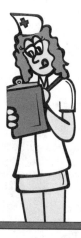

A90

Only answer 3 correctly lists the combination of signs and symptoms that alert the nurse to magnesium sulfate toxicity. Nursing interventions would include immediate discontinuation of the MgSO4 drip, calling for assistance, notifying the physician, and administering calcium gluconate, the antidote medication. Answers 1, 2, and 4 are all incorrect.

Questions

The pediatric nurse explains the schedule of vaccinations to first-time parents. The nurse knows that her clients have understood the information when they reiterate:

1) "We'll return for the DPT, poliomyelitis, and Hib vaccines at 3, 6, and 9 months, and the MMR when the baby is one."
2) "We'll return for the DPT, poliomyelitis, and Hib vaccines at 2, 4, and 6 months, and the MMR when the baby is 9 months."
3) "We'll return for the DPT, poliomyelitis, and Hib vaccines at 2, 4, and 6 months, and the MMR when the baby is one."
4) "We'll return for the MMR at 2, 4, and 6 months, and the poliomyelitis and Hib vaccines when the baby is one."

*Your Own Answer*_____

In order to calculate the correct dose of a medication for a child older than 2 years, the nurse knows that Clark's rule can be used. The equation for Clark's rule is:

1) child's age (years) / child's age + 12 X adult dose = child's dose
2) child's age (years) / child's weight + 12 X adult dose = child's dose
3) child's weight (pounds) / 150 X adult dose = child's dose
4) child's weight (kilograms) / 100 X adult dose = child's dose

*Your Own Answer*_____

Correct Answers

A91

The recommended schedule for infant vaccines is: DPT (diphtheria/pertussis/tetanus), oral poliomyelitis, and Hib *(Haemophilis influenzae* b) at 2, 4, and 6 months, and MMR (measles/mumps/rubella) at one year of age. Therefore, answer 3 is correct and answers 1, 2, and 4 are not.

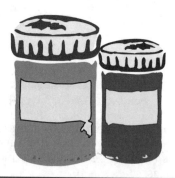

A92

Answer 1 is the equation for Young's rule, and is therefore incorrect. Answers 2 and 4 are also incorrect. Answer 3 is the correct equation for Clark's rule.

Questions

Q93

The nurse is preparing a seven-year-old girl for a tonsillectomy. The most appropriate explanation to this client would be:

1) "The doctor is going to give your throat a boo-boo, but first you'll go to sleepyland so you won't feel anything ouchy."
2) "First you'll get medicine so you can sleep during the operation; then a surgeon will take out the tonsils, so your throat won't get sore anymore."
3) "An anesthesiologist will administer a sedative through an IV; then the surgeon will perform the tonsillectomy."
4) "There is nothing to worry about. You won't feel anything at all, and you'll just sleep and sleep through the operation."

*Your Own Answer*_____

Q94

All of the following could be appropriate nursing diagnoses for the parents with a chronically ill child EXCEPT:

1) potential social isolation related to caring for a frequently hospitalized child
2) self-care deficit related to caring for a chronically hospitalized child
3) potential impaired home management related to caring for an ill child
4) anxiety related to parental role conflict and financial worry and strain

*Your Own Answer*_____

Correct Answers

A93

In answer 1, the nurse uses language too simplistic, as well as condescending, for a child of seven years; this is therefore not the best choice. Answer 3 uses language too sophisticated for a child this age; therefore, this is not a good choice. In answer 4, also a poor choice, the nurse shows a lack of respect for the child's need to understand in simple, concrete terms what is about to happen to her. Furthermore, the implication in this statement to a seven-year-old might be that she will never awaken from the operation. Only answer 2, the best choice, demonstrates the nurse's understanding of the appropriate content and attitude in explaining upcoming surgery to a seven-year-old client.

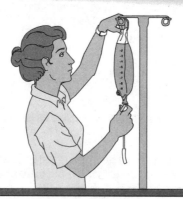

A94

Answer 4, the correct choice, is a psychiatric diagnosis, not a nursing diagnosis. Answers 1, 2, and 3 are all appropriate potential nursing diagnoses for parents with a child who is hospitalized frequently.

Questions

Q95

Jesse is an 11-month-old boy who has been hospitalized since 5 months of age due to a failure to thrive. He has difficulty sitting up unassisted and does not yet attempt to vocalize. His parents visit him most days after work for 3 hours and spend some time with him each weekend. The parents ask the nurse what would be some appropriate gifts to buy Jesse for his first birthday. The nurse's best response would be:

1) a tricycle
2) a rocking horse
3) a jigsaw puzzle
4) board books

*Your Own Answer*_____

Q96

The pediatric nurse is assigned the care of a 3-year-old girl with nephrotic syndrome. The nurse is aware that she will have to assess this client for the following:

1) edema of the extremities, skin breakdown, increased urinary output, and infection
2) generalized edema, skin breakdown, decreased urinary output, and infection
3) generalized edema, skin breakdown, increased urinary output, and hyperactivity
4) abdominal ascites, skin breakdown, muscle twitching, and decreased respirations

*Your Own Answer*_____

Correct Answers

Chronically ill children who spend a fair amount of time in the hospital tend to have developmental delays. Therefore, it is important to focus on the child's developmental age as opposed to his or her chronological age when selecting toys or activities or when interacting. For a child who is not yet sitting unassisted, a tricycle or rocking horse would be inappropriate gifts. Jigsaw puzzles are generally beyond the ability of a developmentally "normal" one-year-old; therefore answer C is a poor choice. Board books, answer D, are a good choice—they usually have large, bold pictures and simple words—and would provide verbal stimulation when read to him by caregivers.

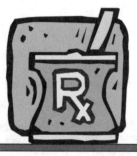

Nephrotic syndrome is the most common form of glomerular injury in children. It consists of massive proteinuria and hypoalbuminema, which cause decreased urinary output, insidious generalized edema and the consequent skin breakdown, leaving the child prone to infection. Answer 2 is therefore correct, and 1, 3, and 4 are all incorrect.

Questions

Q97

Cystic fibrosis is suspected in the child who fails to thrive and/or has duplicate positive sweat chloride tests. The diagnosis is confirmed by which of the following lab values:

1) ≥ 60 mEq/L of sweat chloride content
2) 18 mEq/L of sweat chloride content
3) 20 to 40 mEq/L of sweat chloride content
4) 40 to 60 mEq/L of sweat chloride content

*Your Own Answer*_____

Q98

The nurse teaches families of children with sickle-cell anemia to help their children minimize tissue deoxygenation through all of the following means EXCEPT:

1) avoiding contact sports when spleen is enlarged to protect from potential rupture
2) avoiding all strenuous physical activities, especially those involving running
3) avoiding low-oxygen environments, such as nonpressurized airplane cabins
4) avoiding coming into contact with even mildly infectious individuals

*Your Own Answer*_____

Correct Answers

Normal sweat chloride content is less than 40 mEq/L, with a mean of 18 mEq/L. Sweat chloride content of 40 to 60 is suggestive of cystic fibrosis, with greater than 60 mEq/L being diagnostic. Therefore, answer 1 is correct and 2, 3, and 4 are incorrect.

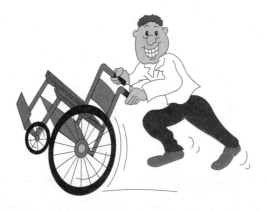

Answers 1, 3, and 4 all make sound recommendations for the protection of the child with sickle-cell anemia from situations that can increase tissue hypoxia, which can lead to tissue necrosis. Therefore, these answers are not the correct choices. It is not necessary to have the child with sickle-cell anemia avoid all physical activity, but it is wise to encourage frequent periods of rest during activity. Therefore, answer 2 is the best choice.

Questions

Q99

The most serious issue surrounding the use of opioid analgesics in the treatment of sickle-cell crisis in children is:

1) the actual likelihood of addiction to these drugs
2) the perceived likelihood of addiction to these drugs
3) their frequent lack of efficacy, no matter the dose
4) all of the above

*Your Own Answer*_____

Q100

The nurse is aware that congenital hip dysplasia can be easily assessed in the newborn by:

1) abducting the hips with the knees and spine flexed—Ortolani's sign is present if a click is heard or felt
2) adducting the hips with the knees and spine flexed—Ortolani's sign is present if grinding is heard
3) abducting the hips with the knees and spine extended—Ortolani's sign is absent if a click is heard or felt
4) adducting the hips with the knees and spine extended—Ortolani's sign is absent if a click is heard or felt

*Your Own Answer*_____

Correct Answers

A99

Opioid analgesics are medically indicated and highly efficacious in the treatment of sickle-cell crisis in children. Less than 1 percent of those receiving opioid analgesics for the severe pain associated with a sickle-cell crisis ever become psychologically dependent on these drugs. Therefore, answers 1, 3, and 4 are not the best choices. The most problematic issue is the perception on the part of parents, as well as health professionals, that addiction is very likely. Consequently, many children with sickle-cell anemia are undermedicated at the time of a crisis. Therefore, answer 2 is correct.

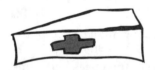

A100

Congenital hip dysplasia is a malformation due to faulty development of the proximal femur. On the affected side, assessment should be for shortening of the leg and asymmetrical skin folds at the thigh and buttocks. A positive Ortolani's sign is diagnostic as well, as correctly described in answer 1. Answers 2, 3, and 4 are all therefore incorrect.

Questions

Mr. Smith has just undergone needle biopsy of his liver which was done as a bedside procedure. Your assessment reveals him to be alert and oriented with stable vital signs. His lungs are clear to auscultation over all fields with an even respiratory rate of eighteen per minute. His abdomen is soft, not tender, and has bowel sounds in all quadrants. An intravenous is infusing at a rate to keep the vein open. The safest activity for Mr. Smith immediately post procedure is:

1) out of bed, ambulating as tolerated
2) bedrest in the right side laying position
3) bedrest in the left side laying position
4) Trendelenberg's position

Your Own Answer

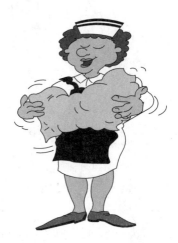

Correct Answers

This question tests your knowledge and ability to maintain safety following an invasive diagnostic procedure through assessment and implementation of nursing care. Answer 1 is incorrect because it is not appropriate for a patient to be ambulating immediately following liver biopsy. Answer 2 is correct. The patient should be maintained for a prescribed period of time on his right side. This position facilitates compression of the liver (which is very vascular) and will aid in the prevention of bleeding and possible hypovolemia, two potential complications of this procedure. Answer 3 is not correct as left side laying offers no particular benefit following liver biopsy. Answer 4 is not correct because elevation of the foot of the bed in a straight tilt is not helpful for this patient. This position was traditionally used to treat shock and encourage blood to the brain but is now quite controversial.

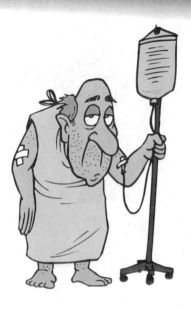

Questions

A male patient returns to the floor one hour after completion of left and right heart catheterization and coronary angiography via the left femoral artery. His condition is stable as he arrives on your floor. His orders require assessment of his vital signs, catheterization site (left groin), measurement of the left lower extremity, and palpation of peripheral pulses every thirty minutes. Two hour mark assessment reveals the following changes: increased left thigh measurement, diminished pedal pulse on left side, left toes cool and dusky in color compared to the right. His left groin dressing is dry and intact. A small drop in blood pressure is noted with an elevated pulse rate. You place a call to the surgeon realizing that these signs may indicate:

1) slow leakage of blood from catheterization site into surrounding tissues resulting in inadequate peripheral blood flow
2) nothing more than preexisting peripheral vascular disease which is noted only upon close assessment of the limb
3) that the patient has developed an arterial thrombi due to hypercoagulation medication administered to minimize bleeding
4) normal and expected post procedure changes which are benign and expected following cardiac catheterization

*Your Own Answer*_____

Correct Answers

This question tests ability to analyze assessment data. Answer 1 is correct as these signs and symptoms may indicate bleeding due to the introduction of a large bore canula into the femoral artery to facilitate this procedure. Pressure dressings and direct pressure immediately following the removal of this instrument are usually successful at controlling bleeding. Depending upon severity of bleeding, life and/or limb may be compromised. Answer 2 is incorrect because these changes were not present during baseline assessments. Answer 3 is not correct as coagulant drugs are not utilized routinely in this procedure. Answer 4 is incorrect as compromise to a distal body site and bleeding significant enough to cause a drop in blood pressure are usually not expected.

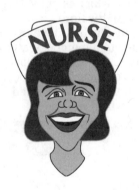

Questions

A newly admitted patient has been ringing her call bell repeatedly for unnecessary requests. Realizing that this patient is exhibiting feelings of anxiety and loss of control, you institute a schedule of visits every fifteen minutes to the patient's room to assess her needs, offer assistance with toileting, and monitor her intravenous fluids. After several hours the patient is noted to be resting quietly when visited and to use the call bell only occasionally. You decide to decrease the frequency of visits to every thirty minutes because this change in the patient's behavior likely reflects:

1) her resignation that her needs cannot be met while she is admitted to this floor as an inpatient
2) her reassurance that the staff is available to assist and support her in her physiological and psychosocial needs
3) the patient's tiring of attention from the staff which she is now avoiding by pretending to nap during visits to her room
4) that this patient's tranquilizer has begun to take effect and she is no longer feeling so anxious

*Your Own Answer*_____

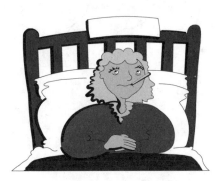

A103

This question focuses upon the evaluation of your plan of care. Answer 1 is incorrect since this is not the goal you were trying to attain and hopefully not what the patient has perceived. Answer 2 is correct as reassurance in this manner is often effective in calming a patient and assisting her to feel more secure in unusual surroundings. Answer 3 is not the correct answer as the patient has been noted to utilize the call bell more appropriately. Answer 4 is incorrect as the change in behavior with appropriate use of the call bell reflects learning rather than oversedation.

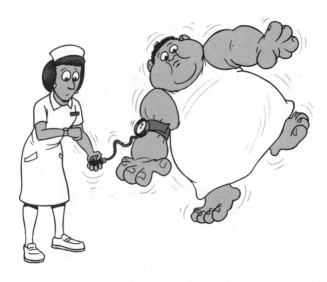

Questions

A young patient has been admitted for observation following a car accident. Many visitors are noted in the room at once with overflow congregating in the hallway outside of his room. The nurse requests that only two visitors at a time remain on the floor and offers that the remainder can wait in a lounge at the end of the hall. The patient becomes angry but is calmed after the nurse explains:

1) his roommate may become jealous of the attention that he is getting from the large quantity of visitors

2) the hallways must be kept clear to prevent injury or delay in the event that an emergency situation should arise

3) his visitors may become ill due to prolonged exposure to the host of germs and bacteria in the air

4) he will be able to visit with his friends and family when he is discharged in twenty-four hours

*Your Own Answer*_____

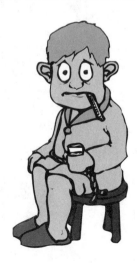

Correct Answers

This question involves implementation of your plan to maintain a safe environment. Answer 1 is incorrect because this is not an appropriate reason to limit visitors to a patient or an appropriate explanation for doing so. If the roommate were disturbed by reasonable visitation, arrangements to visit elsewhere may be arranged. Answer 2 is the correct answer to this question as obstacles, including people, can hinder response time to and/or cause or receive injuries during an emergent situation. Answer 3 is incorrect as this patient needs to visit with his support persons in this time period following trauma. Although physical injury may not be severe, his feelings should be validated as an appropriate response during the posttrauma period.

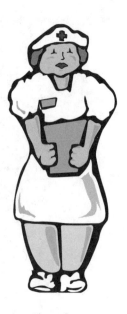

Questions

While administering evening medication, you notice that a patient has a large tube of topical medication, which he has been using for a chronic skin condition for several years, at his bedside. You inform him that all medications must be kept locked in the medication cart and the patient becomes upset. He states he has always administered this medication himself and has never had a problem. The nurse explains that this precaution is necessary because:

1) you fear that he may cause injury to himself by using the medication incorrectly
2) hospital policy strictly requires it of all medications and there are to be no exceptions
3) a patient confused by unfamiliar surroundings may accidentally ingest the medication
4) allowing him to keep it may encourage others to keep medications in their rooms

*Your Own Answer*_____

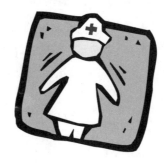

Correct Answers

A105

This question involves the implementation of a plan to maintain environmental safety on the hospital floor. Answer 1 is incorrect as you are sure the patient is capable of continuing self-administration of this medication based upon his history thus far. Answer 2 is not correct as it is not an acceptable rationale for limit setting and will distract from a patient's sense of self worth and autonomy. Answer 3 is the correct answer because it explains a conceivable danger to the patient who may become less upset after processing this information. Answer 4 is incorrect as it does not offer the patient a reassuring rationale for the limit setting.

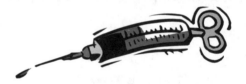

Questions

The nurse has completed her patient teaching modules with Mr. Jones, an elderly man injured by tripping over an object on the floor at home. The nurse knows that outcome criteria promoting environmental safety have been met when the patient verbalizes:

1) "It is important to take my medications about the same time each day."
2) "Each year I will be sure to ask my primary care person if I need a flu shot."
3) "Plenty of fluids and roughage will help to keep bowel elimination regular."
4) "All rooms and floors should be free of clutter and with secured area rugs."

*Your Own Answer*_____

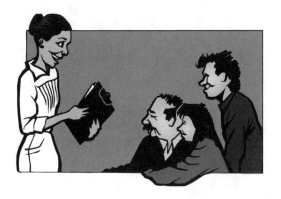

Correct Answers

This question involves evaluation of the efficacy of your implemented plan of care. Answers 1 and 2 are incorrect as they do not relate to environmental safety. Answer 4 is correct because the patient is properly verbalizing material which has been specifically instructed upon to ensure a safe home environment and prevent subsequent falls and injury.

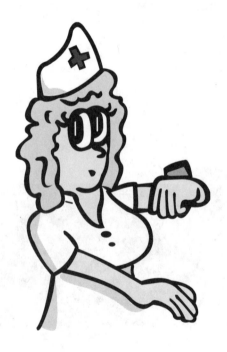

Questions

The nurse is planning to teach a patient with asthma about his medications. He has been prescribed triamcinolone (Azmacort), an inhaled corticosteroid, two puffs twice daily and albuterol sulfate (Proventil), a bronchodilator, two puffs every four hours as needed. The most important fact that the nurse should stress in her teaching is:

1) in order to prevent oral candidiasis, he must be sure to rinse his mouth after each use of bronchodilator

2) use of a bronchodilator, such as albuterol sulfate (Proventil), will help to reduce the amount of future acute asthma attacks

3) only an inhaled corticosteroid like triamcinalone (Azmacort) will offer relief during an acute asthma attack

4) only a fast acting bronchodilator, such as albuterol (Proventil), will give him immediate relief from an acute asthma attack

*Your Own Answer*_____

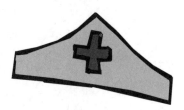

Correct Answers

This question tests your skill at planning teaching goals for the management of a patient with a chronic disease such as asthma. Answer 1 is incorrect. Oral candidiasis can occur from the chronic use of an inhaled corticosteroid steroid, not from a bronchodilator. The patient should be taught to rinse his mouth well following each usage. Answer 2 is not correct because the frequent use of a bronchodilator does not have an impact on the frequency of future asthma attacks. Regular use of an inhaled corticosteroid has been found to decrease the frequency of asthma attacks and the need for rescue doses of bronchodilator. Answer 3 is incorrect. It is essential that patients are instructed that their metered dose inhaler is a maintenance medication and should never be used during an acute attack as it will not cause bronchodilation. For this reason, answer 4 is correct. Many patients find it helpful to label their rapid acting bronchodilator "for acute attack" and their corticosteroid "not for acute attack." This is helpful to the patient and anyone trying to assist them to choose the proper inhaler for relief during an acute event.

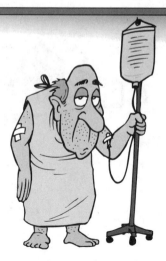

Questions

A patient on your medical-surgical floor has been admitted for treatment of significant cirrhosis of the liver. Insertion of a portal-caval shunt is being considered to decrease portal hypertension. His skin and sclera are icteric. He is weak but, upon admission, his vital signs are stable. Assessing his vital signs prior to administration of evening medications you note a drop in his blood pressure and an increased pulse rate which is thready in quality. He is increasingly weak and diaphoretic. He tells you he is nauseated and that he feels as though he may vomit. Following this assessment the nurse should:

1) call the house officer and obtain a standing order for an antiemetic medication to relive nausea and prevent vomiting
2) offer the patient a glass of flat, room temperature ginger ale in the hope that it will settle his upset stomach
3) suspect bleeding esophageal varices and monitor him closely while summoning the house physician and placing a call to the physician
4) suspect that the patient is constipated and prepare to administer a high colonic enema in order to provide the patient some relief

Your Own Answer_____

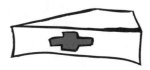

Correct Answers

This question tests your ability to assess a patient with a chronic disease and analyze obtained data to recognize what may be an acute or emergent problem. Answer 1 is not the correct answer. Administration of an antiemetic would only mask some of the symptoms which when clustered with other assessment data such as hypotension, diaphoresis, and increasing weakness suggests the onset of an emergent situation which requires intervention. Similarly answer 2 is not correct as it does not address the possibility of serious complications which may be beginning. Answer 3 is correct. The nurse recognizes that the patient may have bleeding esophageal varices as a result of sustained portal hypertension and that this situation is potentially life threatening. She also knows that this complication requires immediate intervention (fluid resuscitation, iced saline lavage, direct pressure to the bleeding site) and closely monitors the patient while waiting for assistance. Answer 4 is incorrect. It is contraindicated to administer an enema of any kind without explicit orders from the physician to any patient with liver disease. A patient with portal hypertension is likely to have extensive hemorrhoids which may bleed if disturbed. Impaired liver function may also impair the synthesis of clotting factors normally produced in this organ which may complicate hemostasis and make clotting difficult.

Questions

A nineteen-year-old female patient just seen at the ambulatory clinic was diagnosed with acute cystitis. She has been prescribed a sulfonamide antibiotic containing sulfamethoxazole 800mg and trimethoprim 160 mg (Bactrim DS) to be taken twice daily. The nurse instructs the patient to:

1) limit her fluid intake while she is taking this medication
2) take this medication only with milk to ensure best absorption
3) stop taking this medication as soon as her symptoms subside
4) avoid sun exposure while being treated with this medication

*Your Own Answer*_____

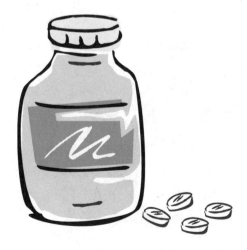

Correct Answers

This question involves the management of an acute illness with a focus on implementation of your patient teaching plan. Answer 1 is incorrect because patients with cystitis need to be encouraged to drink plenty of fluids to aid in flushing bacteria out of the urinary tract, as well as assisting the body to eliminate metabolized drug. Answer 2 is not correct as this statement is not true. The absorption of certain medications is hindered when taken with milk. Answer 3 is incorrect. Antibiotics should be taken for the entire length of time prescribed unless otherwise directed by the primary care provider. This will ensure that all microorganisms are eradicated by the medication thus preventing recurrence of infection and reducing the risk of creating resistant strains of bacteria. Answer 4 is correct. Most sulpha drugs cause significant photosensitivity in those who are taking them. A sunblock should be worn and prolonged exposure to the sun should be avoided.

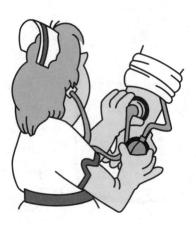

Questions

Mrs. Smith is two days postoperative from bowel surgery that has left her with a transverse colostomy. She is tolerating sips of clear fluids and has intravenous hydration. You place a call to the surgeon after noticing which of the following during ostomy care:

1) the stoma is a pink to red color similar to that of the buccal mucosa
2) a small amount of foul smelling mushy drainage is noted in the ostomy bag
3) the stoma is noted to be a dark red to dusky blue color upon assessment
4) the stoma protrudes slightly from the abdomen and is somewhat swollen

Your Own Answer

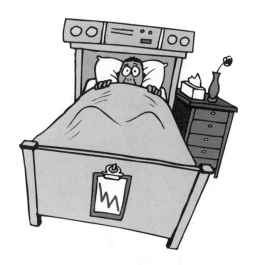

Correct Answers

This question tests your knowledge of care appropriate for a patient following an acute surgical procedure. Focus is upon assessment and analysis of data collected. Answer 1 is not the correct answer as this describes a normal finding and will not require any urgent interventions. Answer 2 is incorrect because this, too, is to be expected in a patient with a transverse colostomy and also confirms that bowel function has returned postoperatively. This indicates that, physiologically, the patient is recovering well from the trauma of abdominal surgery. Absence of ostomy function and bowel sounds might indicate the complication of paralytic ileus. Answer 3 is the correct answer to this question. The nurse recognizes that this may describe a stoma with compromised vascularity and may require surgical intervention. Answer 4 is incorrect. Stomas normally tend to protrude slightly from the abdomen. It is also normal for new stomas to have some degree of swelling which can be expected to subside over a period of two to four weeks postoperatively.

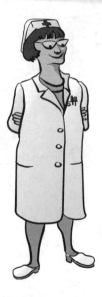

Questions

Mr. Adams is admitted to your medical-surgical floor for an exacerbation of his chronic obstructive pulmonary disease (COPD) with a mild to moderate degree of hypoxia. His plan of care incorporates mucolytics and expectorants to aid in thinning and expectoration of respiratory secretions. He is also placed on an antibiotic to fight any infectious process which may be contributory to his exacerbation. He is on oxygen at three liters per minute via nasal cannula. His regimen seems to improve his status and Mr. Adams is noted to be breathing more easily. A visiting family member requests that his oxygen flow rate be increased to provide further relief of dyspnea. As his primary nurse, what is your response to this request:

1) call the physician to obtain an order to increase the oxygen flow rate
2) tell the family member to adjust the flow rate for the patient's comfort
3) explain that increasing oxygen flow rate would not be appropriate
4) place a call to the respiratory therapist to request additional oxygen supplies

*Your Own Answer*_____

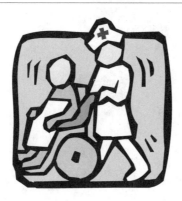

Correct Answers

A111

This question tests management skill for this chronic disease process through data analysis and knowledgeable planning of care. Answer 1 is incorrect, as are answers 2 and 4. Patients with COPD undergo physiologic changes due to chronically elevated levels of carbon dioxide. In a healthy patient, these high levels of carbon dioxide trigger the action of breathing whereby carbon dioxide is expelled or "blown off" in exchange for oxygen. In the patient with COPD, carbon dioxide levels are chronically elevated and the body adapts by using dropping levels of oxygen as the trigger for respiration. If excess oxygen levels were administered to a patient with COPD, he would lose his respiratory stimulus and could potentially stop breathing. This phenomenon is observed at low flow rates of oxygen over two or three liters per minute. This rationale explains why answer 3 is the correct answer to this question. It is essential that patients and family members are educated in order to prevent complications due to good intentions.

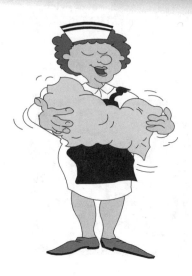

Questions

Q112

Tom, a twenty-five-year-old white male with a long history of epilepsy controlled by antiseizure medication, presents to the ambulatory clinic. He states he is generally not feeling well and has been slightly dizzy since this morning. While registering to be seen he suddenly lets out a strange grunt, falls to the floor, and begins to exhibit generalized tonic and clonic movements. The nurse, reacting quickly:

1) knows that Tom is experiencing a grand mal seizure and turns him onto his side as she calls for assistance
2) suspects a petit mal seizure and attempts to insert a pen between clenched teeth to preserve his airway
3) attempts to pour orange juice into his mouth to increase his glucose levels and correct hypoglycemia
4) recognizes a focal motor seizure and attempts to immobilize the involved areas of the body

*Your Own Answer*_____

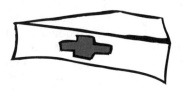

Correct Answers

This question pertains to management of a chronic disease process which presents as an emergent situation. Answer 1 is correct as the patient's history and description of his condition are consistent with the grand mal seizure common in epilepsy. A grunt may immediately precede the onset of seizure activity as air is forced out of the lungs. The nurse is correct in turning the patient on his side (or in "the recovery position") which facilitates the drainage of secretions or emesis from his oral cavity and preservation of the airway. All hard, pointed, or otherwise hazardous objects should be moved out of the patient's surrounding to prevent further injury. Answer 2 is incorrect. The presented data is not consistent with a petit mal (or "absence") seizure which involves brief periods where the patient loses consciousness and seems to "tune out." There are no corresponding motor signs or symptoms and often the patient is not aware of the episode(s). No objects should be inserted into the mouth of a patient experiencing a seizure. Forcing an object through clenched teeth and jaw may push the tongue toward the back of the oropharynx and cause airway occlusion. (Again, clenched teeth and jaw do not occur with a petit mal seizure.) Answer 3 is incorrect. Seizures due to hypoglycemia do occur but the presented data and history are not consistent with this scenario. No liquid should be forced into the mouth of any patient with an altered level of consciousness. Answer 4 is incorrect. A focal motor seizure does not necessarily involve the loss of consciousness nor involvement of the entire body. Involved areas should be protected from injury but not forcefully immobilized.

Questions

Ms. Jones arrives at the emergency department. Her face and eyes are red and swollen. She is covered with a diffuse blotchy rash and she has difficulty breathing and speaking due to shortness of breath and wheezing. Vital signs reveal hypotension (blood pressure of 85/50) and tachycardia (pulse rate of 130 beats per minute). A friend accompanying her states they had just left the restaurant where they had eaten dinner when symptoms began. Ms. Jones is reported to be in good health with no medical problems. She is on no medications and without drug allergy. She has a history of allergy to pine nuts. The nurse prepares to administer:

1) a tranquilizer to relieve this patient who is obviously suffering from effects of a severe anxiety attack
2) an antithrombolytic to prevent permanent damage resulting from this acute myocardial infarction
3) a narcotic antagonist drug to reverse the effects which are occurring from an overdose of narcotics
4) epinephrine, a sympathomimetic, to treat the anaphylactic reaction that this patient is encountering

*Your Own Answer*_____

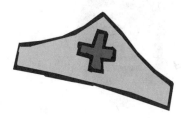

Correct Answers

This question involves analysis of provided data in an emergency situation. Answer 4 is the correct answer. Presenting signs and symptoms and history are consistent with this severe allergic reaction, which was probably caused by undetected ingestion of the pine nuts to which this patient is allergic. Ingredients in salad dressings, sauces, and other foods can trigger reactions to foods which are "disguised" and unknowingly ingested when they are blended or chopped in a recipe. Anaphylaxis can have a rapid onset and quickly become fatal due to resultant shock, circulatory collapse, and edema of the airways. Answer 1 is incorrect as edema would not usually occur with an anxiety attack. Answer 2 is incorrect. No information has been presented to indicate that this woman is suffering an acute myocardial infarction. Facial edema, wheezing, and skin rash are not consistent with this hypothesis. Answer 3 is incorrect as we have not received any information to indicate that this patient has overdosed on narcotics. Presentation is consistent with severe allergic reaction. In the emergency room, however, drug abuse is frequently in the differential diagnosis and would be more strongly considered should the patient fail to respond to primary treatment.

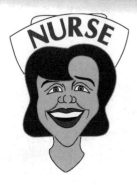

Questions

Ms. Smith is a forgetful elderly female with multiple chronic medical problems. She has required specialist care for various aspects of her management including chronic obstructive pulmonary disease (COPD), diabetes, and hypertension. She often cannot recall the names or dosages of medications which have been changed or added by a specialist. The specialists are not always available and consultation reports may take several weeks to be received by the primary care provider. You know your patient teaching has been successful when she arrives for her appointment with:

1) copies of old hospital instructions stating medications and treatment regimens which she was discharged on over the past five years
2) her new home health aide who reminds her to take medications which are prepoured by the visiting nurse each week
3) a notebook containing names and dosages of current medications and weekly blood sugars prepared by the visiting nurse
4) her medication holder which contains her multiple medications which are prepoured for her by a neighbor

*Your Own Answer*_____

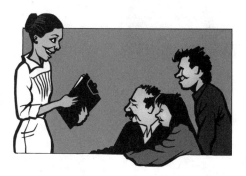

Correct Answers

This question involves the evaluation of your implemented plan for a patient with multiple chronic disease processes. Ms. Smith was instructed through teaching and written information (to be reviewed by her visiting nurse). This multidisciplinary approach has finally impressed the importance of having a primary care coordinator who is current with her medications and treatments. This is exhibited in the correct answer to this question, answer 3, which involves the patient's maintenance of a record to be updated during each visit to a care giver. This decreases the chance of the patient forgetting instructions and can serve as a reminder to enhance compliance at home. Answer 1 is not correct as this information is not current. Answers 2 and 4 are not correct as prepoured medications are difficult to identify.

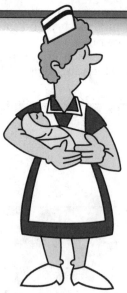

Questions

Mrs. Jones is admitted to the hospital after being diagnosed as suffering a cerebral vascular accident (CVA). This event has left her with a right hemiparesis. In planning her care to prevent complications due to immobility the nurse:

1) obtains an order for a low fat, low protein, low calorie diet to prevent weight gain while inactive
2) arranges for the delivery of books and television installation to encourage the patient to maintain bedrest
3) obtains an order for a foley catheter so the patient will not need to be moved for toileting
4) institutes a regimen of turning and positioning and regular skin assessment for redness or breaks in skin

*Your Own Answer*_____

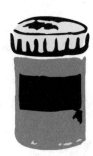

Correct Answers

A115

This question involves prevention of complications due to what could become chronic immobility. Answer 1 is incorrect. A patient needs a diet with adequate protein, nutrients, and calories to support healing. A dietary consultation may be in order. Answer 2 is the incorrect answer as this suggestion will increase risk of pressure ulcer formation, atelectasis, and muscle atrophy. Answer 3 is incorrect. It is inappropriate to insert an indwelling urinary catheter to avoid moving a patient. Unnecessary use may lead to the complication of urinary tract infection. Answer 4 is the correct answer to this question as it promotes prevention of skin breakdown. Frequent turning and positioning also helps to avoid atelectasis via positional drainage and avoidance of compression of body weight upon one lung (which prevents optimal expansion and may lead to respiratory complications).

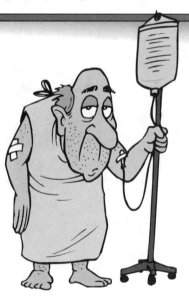

Questions

Q116

Tara is a twenty-three-year-old white female who had her appendix removed early this morning due to acute appendicitis. She has no medical problems except some mild asthma. It is essential to teach Tara what during the early recovery period?

1) be sure to drink large amounts of fluids to prevent dehydration
2) use the bedpan rather than beginning to ambulate too soon
3) splint her incision, take deep breaths, and cough each hour
4) avoid eating foods with high sodium and saturated fat

*Your Own Answer*_____

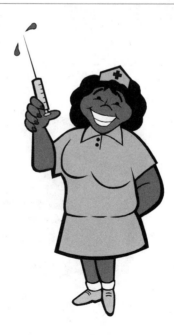

Correct Answers

This question relates to avoiding complications due to surgery and a chronic disease entity. Answer 1 is incorrect. This patient is less than twenty four hours postoperative from abdominal surgery and must begin taking fluids as prescribed by the surgeon, typically in small and frequent amounts to avoid gas pains and nausea and/or vomiting. Answer 2 is incorrect. Early ambulation (as ordered) is important to encourage return of normal gastrointestinal motility and prevent pooling of secretions in the lungs which may lead to pneumonia. Answer 3 is correct and must be encouraged early in the postoperative recovery period as previously explained. Splinting of the incision site helps to make coughing and deep breathing less uncomfortable. Answer 4 is incorrect. These dietary restrictions are not specific to this patient or to the procedure she has undergone.

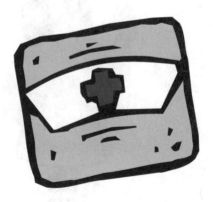

Questions

Q117

Mrs. Jones comes in for a routine physical exam by her primary care provider. She had a right-sided radical mastectomy three years ago for Stage II breast cancer. The nurse knows that post-mastectomy teaching needs reinforcement when she notices:

1) short fingernails which are well cared for with healthy appearing cuticles
2) antecubital ecchymosis on the right arm due to a recent venipuncture
3) a tattoo in the right wrist identified by the patient as ten years old
4) the right arm is mildly edematous but pink in color with a strong radial pulse

Your Own Answer_____

Q118

Many patients with asthma can identify certain trigger factors which may bring on an acute attack. Which of the following is likely to trigger such an episode:

1) covering the nose and mouth with a scarf before going outside in cold weather
2) regular damp dusting in order to keep environmental dust at a minimum
3) spending extended periods of time with pets at a friend's home
4) using an inhaled corticosteroid at least twice daily with a spacer unit attached

Your Own Answer_____

Correct Answers

A117

This question tests your ability to evaluate your plan. Answer 2 is the correct answer and alerts the nurse that teaching needs reinforcement regarding appropriate precautions which need to be undertaken to ensure the integrity of the right limb. Radical mastectomy and/or lymph node dissection leaves lymphatic drainage pathways impaired and, thus, even small breaks in the skin can introduce enough bacteria to cause a serious infection and/or abscess formation. Answer 1 is incorrect since it illustrates the proper care of hands and nails following mastectomy. Intact skin and cuticles are the body's best defense against infection. A tattoo placed on the body prior to the procedure is not dangerous to the limb and therefore answer 3 is wrong. Answer 4 is not the correct answer. Lymphedema, in varying degrees, is experienced by many patients post mastectomy due to impaired lymphatic drainage. It does not reflect that a patient is improperly caring for themselves.

A118

This question deals with preventing complications of a chronic disease. Answer 1 is incorrect seeing as warmed air, unlike cold air, is not likely to trigger bronchospasm. Answer 2 is incorrect. Damp dusting will remove excess dust and dust mites (common asthma irritants) in the home environment. Answer 3 is the correct answer to this question. Animal proteins, from both dander and saliva, are often major asthma triggers. Answer 4 is incorrect because regular use of inhaled corticosteroids helps to reduce frequency of asthma attacks experienced by an individual.

Questions

Mrs. Jones is seen in the office today for a physical exam. She has hypertension and tells you she is worried about developing heart disease. Which of Mrs. Jones' following risk factors for cardiac disease cannot be modified?

1) Her mother had her first myocardial infarction at age 50.
2) Mrs. Jones has been smoking one pack of cigarettes per day.
3) She has been thirty pounds overweight for about ten years.
4) Her cholesterol and triglycerides are significantly elevated.

*Your Own Answer*_____

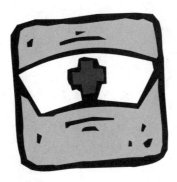

Correct Answers

A119

This question deals with planning and implementing strategies to assist clients in lowering their risk of developing serious health problems. This question stresses the fact that risk of cardiac disease is dramatically reducible through lifestyle modification. Answer 1 is the correct answer to this question. Hereditary risk factors cannot be changed. They should serve as an impetus to aggressively modify those factors that can be changed. Answer 2 is not the correct answer. Smoking raises the risk of heart disease by causing vasoconstriction and thus hypertension may ensue. Nicotine may cause cardiac excitability. Answer 3 is incorrect as, once again, obesity is a modifiable risk factor. Similarly, hyperlipidemia can be controlled via diet, exercise, and medication (if needed) and therefore, answer 4 is not correct.

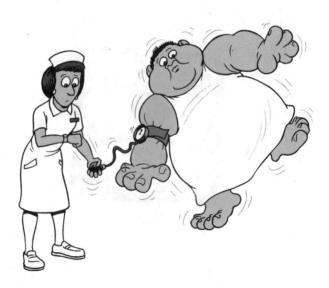

Questions

Jennie is a nineteen-year-old female who presents to the family planning clinic requesting to be put on oral contraceptives. She was treated for pelvic inflammatory disease approximately six months ago. She is G2P0A2. Her most recent elective abortion procedure was one month ago. In planning her patient teaching, you want to stress facts that will promote safe behaviors and decrease Jennie's risk of again becoming pregnant or contracting a sexually transmitted disease. You know that Jennie needs further teaching when she tells you:

1) "Oral contraceptives are effective alone against pregnancy."
2) "A condom can prevent the spread of HIV and other sexually transmitted diseases."
3) "Pelvic infections can cause scarring which may decrease future fertility."
4) "Abstinence is the only 100 percent effective method against pregnancy and disease."

*Your Own Answer*_____

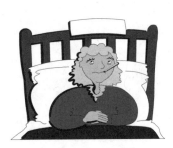

Correct Answers

A120

This question deals with planning care to help patients learn to reduce their risk of disease and health complications. Answer 1 is the correct answer because it may indicate that this client needs further teaching because there is no mention that oral contraceptives offer no protection against sexually transmitted diseases. Answers 2, 3, and 4 are not the correct answers to this question. Each statement offers a fact about sexual health and contraception and is self-explanatory.

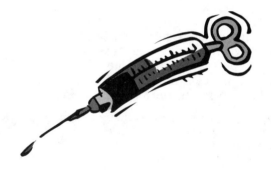

Questions

Joe has a hiatal hernia which has not been problematic or required medication for several years. He now reports severe "heartburn" which gets worse when he lies down. Updating his history, you notice that he has gained twenty pounds. You counsel him on the importance of eating small frequent meals, avoiding spicy food and caffeine, and remaining upright after a meal. You advise him that a serious complication that may occur from a large hiatal hernia is:

1) painful bulging of the hernia upon straining to lift heavy objects at work
2) dependence upon medications to control or neutralize acid production
3) strangulation of the portion of the stomach protruding into the chest cavity
4) the inability to sleep unless sitting upright in a chair to prevent pain

*Your Own Answer*_____

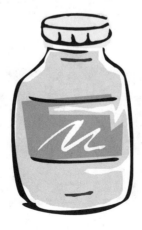

Correct Answers

This question deals with teaching the patient to avoid the risks associated with a chronic condition. Answer 1 is incorrect as a hiatal hernia usually does not bulge with lifting heavy objects. Answer 2 is incorrect as it is unusual for a patient to become addicted to antacids and acid blocking medications. Answer 3 is correct as it identifies a serious complication which may occur from an unmanaged hiatal hernia. This risk increases with obesity, consumption of large meals, and wearing tight clothes. These actions increase the upward pressure on the stomach and force the hernia to slide through the weakness in the diaphragm into the chest cavity. If the stomach becomes strangulated, or "stuck," in this position, serious complications can ensue such as necrosis to the stomach tissues. This may require immediate surgical intervention. Answer 4 is incorrect. Patients with hiatal hernia may experience discomfort when laying down immediately after a meal. Patients are often encouraged to elevate the head of the bed to discourage reflux into the esophagus.

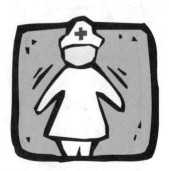

Questions

A sixty-five-year-old female comes in for follow-up assessment and laboratory work for her chronic pernicious anemia. The patient states that although she is feeling well, she continues to tire easily. Which of the following suggestions would this patient find useful?

1) Try to get all of your errands run in the morning and early afternoon so that you have the remainder of the day to rest.
2) Give up all unnecessary obligations such as those involving unimportant groups like senior citizens or the Women's Club.
3) Plan your day with frequent rest periods while you are still fatiguing easily.
4) Complete the series of four injections to treat your anemia and prevent fatigue.

*Your Own Answer*_____

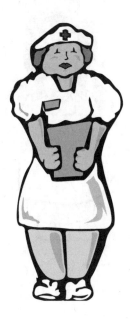

Correct Answers

This question deals with modification of activities of daily living to best fulfill the demands of daily activity. Answer 1 is incorrect because this suggestion will only serve to exhaust the patient and does nothing to aid her in coping with her activities of daily living (ADLs). Answer 2 is incorrect as it does not offer a suggestion which will help the patient accomplish her daily tasks. It is important for a patient to maintain contact with peers if possible during a period of illness. Peer support may help the patient to cope better and avoid depression resulting from her need to alter her usual routine at this time. Answer 3 is the correct answer to this question. Pacing her activity and providing for rest periods may help the patient to accomplish her ADL's with minimal distress. Answer 4 is incorrect. Patients with pernicious anemia require lifelong intramuscular supplementation of Vitamin B12.

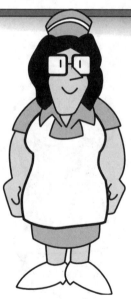

Questions

Mr. Jones is an elderly patient on your unit who is preparing for discharge after being treated for an acute episode of congestive heart disease. While administering his morning medications you notice his menu selections for the next day. You know your patient teaching plan for preventing further acute episodes has been effective when you see that he has chosen:

1) bacon and egg on a roll, tomato juice, and an orange for breakfast
2) chicken noodle soup, crackers, sugar-free gelatin, and a salad for lunch
3) a hamburger, french fries, dill pickle, and a diet cola for dinner
4) oatmeal, egg white omelet, orange juice, and coffee for breakfast

*Your Own Answer*_____

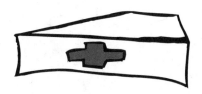

Correct Answers

This question allows you to evaluate your implemented plan teaching a patient with congestive heart failure to avoid an acute exacerbation. A major issue is fluid volume which often becomes overloaded with excessive sodium intake. Patients should be instructed not to add salt at the table, avoid canned foods, and read labels carefully paying attention to portion size. Answer 1 is incorrect. This selection contains too much sodium and fat for a cardiac patient on a sodium restriction. Answer 2 is incorrect as once again there is excessive sodium. Some canned soups contain up to 800 mg of sodium per one cup serving and diet colas can contain about 100 mg per serving depending on the brand. Answer 3 is incorrect and does not reflect planning by the patient for a low-sodium diet. Answer 4 is a reasonable and healthy choice for this patient, assuming that the hospital is serving decaffeinated coffee on a cardiac floor.

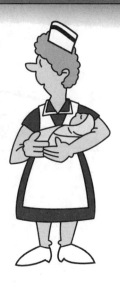

Questions

Q124

John is an avid fisherman. He presents to the office today for routine visit and you notice that he has a deep tan with lots of flat macular pigmented lesions over his shoulders and scalp (he has a significant area of male pattern balding). While assessing his vital signs you:

1) joke that his cholesterol must be lowered from all of the fish he has been eating
2) ask him if his stress level has decreased from enjoying his time fishing
3) advise that he begin to only fish during the evening hours to avoid sun exposure
4) encourage him to wear sunblock, a hat, long sleeves, and sunglasses in the sun

*Your Own Answer*_____

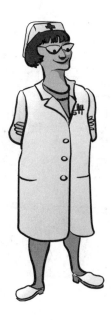

Correct Answers

A124

This question concerns analysis of data from assessment and plan implementation to help a patient prevent future health risks. Answer 1 is incorrect because it does not offer any risk prevention advice related to your brief visual assessment of prolonged sun exposure. Answer 2 is also incorrect for the same reason. Answer 3 is incorrect as it may not be a practical option for this patient and may even increase his risk of physical injury from fishing in the darkness. Answer 4 is correct. Taking measures to avoid overexposure to the sun is vital to preventing the development of skin cancers. This patient should also be advised to have skin assessments at least annually by a health professional and be instructed in self-examination.

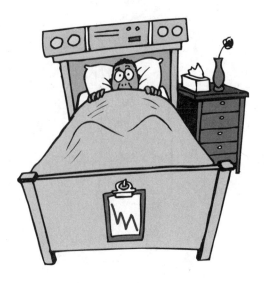

Questions

A twenty-one-year-old white female comes in to the office planning to request a breast exam and a mammogram referral. She has two maternal aunts and a sister with breast cancer and is very anxious that she, too, will contract the disease. During your time with the patient, which of the following is least appropriate?

1) validate this client's feelings of anxiety and encourage her to verbalize her concerns and questions
2) encourage the patient to avoid a diet high in fat which is believed to be associated with breast cancer
3) tell her there is nothing she can do to avoid getting this disease process if she is genetically predisposed to it
4) have her discuss breast ultrasound and/or the early institution of mammogram screening with the physician

*Your Own Answer*_____

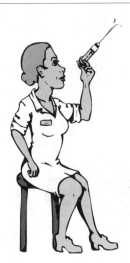

Correct Answers

A125

This question deals with prevention of a disease for which the client may have an increased hereditary risk. Answer 1 is incorrect since this is an important intervention for this client. The nurse can help to empower this young woman to take responsibility for her preventive health care and disease screening. Answer 2 is not the correct answer as this suggestion may be helpful in disease prevention. Answer 3 is the correct answer because this is not an approach to take when promoting early detection of a disease. Women at an increased risk should feel that they are armed with new research and technology in early detection of this disease which has a 90% cure rate (when discovered in situ without lymph node involvement). Answer 4 is not the correct answer because this is an important point to stress. Preventive screening in a high risk individual may differ from the general population. This must be decided on an individual basis and may vary from case to case. Mammograms are not as useful screening tools in young women because increased breast density does not allow the degree of visualization that is obtained in the older women who have less density and elasticity in their breasts. An ultrasound may be useful in younger women.

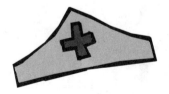

Questions

Jane is on chronic glucocorticoid suppressive therapy for the treatment of asthma. She is maintained on 10 mg of Prednisone daily. You instruct Jane on the signs and symptoms of potential side effects of this medication which may include all <u>but</u> which of the following:

1) increased susceptibility for developing infection
2) increased risk of developing diabetes mellitus
3) varying degrees of weight gain and bloating
4) marked drowsiness and sleep enhancement

*Your Own Answer*_____

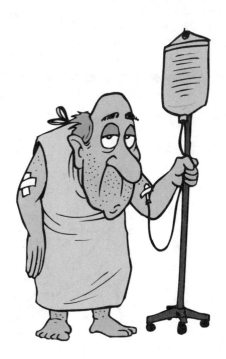

Correct Answers

This question stresses teaching patients to notice the earliest signs and symptoms which may occur while taking medication that increases the risk of developing medical complications. Answer 1 is not the correct answer to this question as this drug works systemically to reduce inflammation which includes the beneficial inflammatory response to invading bacteria or injury. Answer 2 is incorrect. This medication reduces glucose tolerance and may cause the onset of diabetes. Patients should be advised to be alert to polyphagia, polydipsia, and polyuria. Answer 3 is not the correct answer to this question. This steroid causes sodium and water retention which may cause significant weight gain and bloating, especially characteristic are the "moon face" and "buffalo hump." Finally, answer 4 is the correct answer because this statement is false. Steroids don't enhance sleep or promote drowsiness but can often cause an increase in energy and almost "euphoria" in patients taking them.

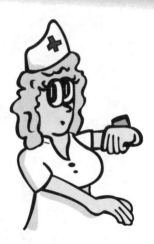

Questions

Mrs. Studdert had a hysterectomy at age thirty-two. She is now sixty and has never been on hormone replacement therapy, so she is sent for bone density testing. Results confirm that she has moderate demineralization at the hip and lumbar spine. The physician places her on Alendronate (Fosamax) 10 mg po daily. You teach her that this medication will need to be taken thirty minutes prior to eating breakfast (on an empty stomach) with a full glass of water. Mrs. Studdert can expect to:

1) discontinue her calcium supplement while she is taking this medication
2) regain the inch and three quarters that she's lost due to compression fractures
3) maintain her current bone density mass without further demineralization
4) find significant relief of her long standing osteoarthritis symptoms

*Your Own Answer*_____

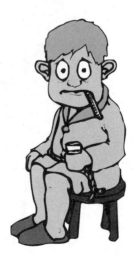

Correct Answers

This question seeks to reduce the risk of complications that may occur due to osteoporosis through analysis of data and plan implementation. The complications of osteoporosis can be devastating and may include pain, severe spinal deformity and kyphosis, pathological fractures (especially of the hip and spine), loss of height (due to spinal compression fractures), activity avoidance, immobility, and a host of other resulting sequelae. Answer 1 is not the correct answer. Adequate calcium intake is still required for women on this medication. Answer 2 is incorrect and is not a realistic expectation. Research now shows that this drug may be able to promote significant remineralization of osteopenic bone as well as prevent further bone density loss. The correct answer is 3 for the reasons just detailed. Answer 4 is an incorrect statement as these benefits have not been found.

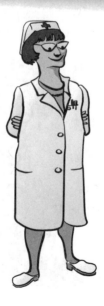

Questions

When providing patient teaching to promote proper management of a patient with chronic iron deficiency anemia, it is best to recommend:

1) taking an iron supplement with an antacid to avoid stomach upset
2) taking a daily iron supplement with a glass of orange juice
3) avoid green leafy vegetables and other roughage
4) disregarding constipation as it is probably not related to iron supplements

*Your Own Answer*_____

Mr. Jones, an eighty-year-old-male, shares with his nurse that his vision is declining and he is upset because he loves to read. The ophthalmologist states that the patient's visual deficit is uncorrectable. The best response of the nurse is to:

1) offer to read to the patient
2) tell him to start watching the soap operas on television
3) obtain large print and talking books for the patient
4) say nothing using therapeutic pause to explore feelings

*Your Own Answer*_____

Correct Answers

A128

This question involves planning and implementation to prevent a chronic disease from becoming acute through patient education. Iron deficiency anemia is commonly treated with oral iron supplementation along with dietary modifications. Answer 1 is incorrect as antacids will considerably reduce the amount of iron absorbed in the stomach. Answer 2 is correct. Orange juice has been found to enhance the absorption of supplemental iron. Answer 3 is incorrect as green leafy vegetables are a good source of dietary iron. Roughage intake will aid in the management of constipation. Answer 4 is incorrect. Patients for whom iron supplementation is prescribed must be warned of the possibility of constipation and methods by which they can manage the same. It should be noted that constipation is a common reason that patients are not compliant with iron supplementation regimens.

A129

This question focuses on promotion of activities of daily living through modification for a disability. Answer 1 is incorrect. The patient is upset over an inevitable decline in his independence. Answer 2 is not correct, either, as Mr. Jones would probably not relate to daytime television as he does to his classic books. Answer 3 is the correct answer to this question. These modifications will promote self-esteem in this patient who is slowly experiencing a loss of function. Answer 4 is incorrect, but might be helpful to explore feelings should the patient give signals he wishes to verbalize.

Questions

A seventy-year-old-male type I diabetic has been managing his disease well (with a hemoglobin AIC of 7.0) through dietary modification and the administration of 28 units of Humulin 70/30 insulin. Lately he has had a decline in his vision due to deficits caused by uncorrectable diabetic retinopathy. He reports that it is becoming more difficult to read the unit number markings on the U-100 insulin syringe that he uses. Which of the following would not be a viable option:

1) arrange for a visiting nurse to visit weekly and prefill his syringes for him
2) teach him how to utilize a magnification device designed for insulin syringes
3) instruct one of his family members in properly drawing up insulin into a syringe
4) have his physician discontinue his insulin and begin oral hypoglycemic therapy

Your Own Answer_____

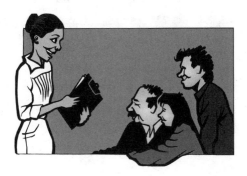

Correct Answers

This question examines planning and implementation skills. Diabetic retinopathy affects up to 90 percent of patients with diabetes after twenty years of disease. Fortunately, total blindness will occur only in a small percentage of patients with this chronic complication. Answer 1 is not the correct answer because it presents a realistic solution to the progressive disability of this patient and does not compromise the treatment plan. Also incorrect is answer 2 because it might enable the patient to continue on his medication regimen independent of outside assistance. A variety of magnification type devices are available and have been helpful to many individuals. Answer 3, again, presents a workable plan to promote continuity of this patient's plan of care in combination with some assistance from a reliable family member and is therefore not the correct answer. Answer 4 is the correct answer to this question. Attempting glycemic control via the use of an oral hypoglycemic agent is not a viable option. Oral hypoglycemic agents stimulate pancreatic islets to release insulin into the blood stream inducing the lowering of serum glucose levels. Type I diabetic patients are unable to manufacture insulin and for this reason, this type of drug will have no impact upon glycemic control.

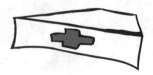

Questions

Mrs. Jones has been diagnosed with diverticulosis. After instructing her in dietary management, you teach her to be alert for signs and symptoms of an acute attack of diverticulitis which includes fever in combination with all but which of the following:

1) weakness and fatigue
2) left lower quadrant pain
3) narrow stools
4) frequent urination

Your Own Answer

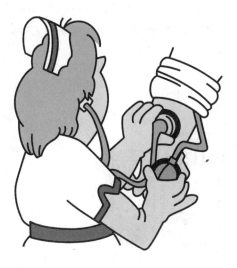

Correct Answers

This question involves planning and implementation. An acute attack of diverticulitis can lead to perforation of the bowel, peritonitis, and even death in severe cases. Educating the patient to be alert for signs of trouble is important to health maintenance/prevention of complications. Answer 1 in combination with fever should signal the patient that she may be harboring a chronic inflammation of the involved segment of the large bowel or developing an acute infection of the same, making this an incorrect answer to this question. This may occur when fecal material collects in the characteristic outpouching of the bowel. Answer 2 is also incorrect. Diverticula commonly occur in the sigmoid area of the large intestine and would create tenderness in the left lower quadrant of the abdomen should it become inflamed. Answer 3 is not the correct answer because narrow stools may occur due to inflammation and edema in the affected area of bowel. Answer 4 is the correct answer as frequent urination is not usually a symptom of diverticulitis.

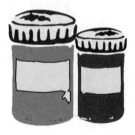

Questions

Q132

Eighty-five-year-old Mary Jones has been diagnosed with gallbladder calculi (of cholesterol origin) after an attack of fever, diarrhea, and right upper quadrant abdominal pain. She has been deemed a poor surgical candidate due to other chronic health problems. She has responded well to antibiotic therapy and the health care team has decided to attempt management through use of diet/lifestyle modification and pharmacotherapy with chenodeoxycholic acid. What will you teach Ms. Jones not to do?

1) avoid fatty foods such as cream, fried foods, and cheeses
2) begin attempts to promote the loss of excess body weight
3) report the occurrence of any fever, chills, or abdominal pain
4) take her medication only when she is having abdominal tenderness

*Your Own Answer*_____

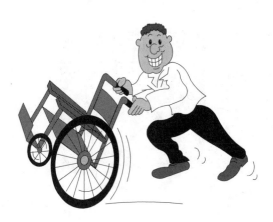

Correct Answers

This question deals with avoiding risks associated with chronic disease. In this case, the patient's chronic disease puts her at risk of serious infection and possibly peritonitis due to her judged inability to survive a surgical procedure. Answer 1 is not the correct answer as Ms. Jones must avoid fatty/high cholesterol foods to avoid the irritating effect of their metabolites when excreted into the gallbladder and/or the formation of further calculi. Answer 2 is not the correct answer because obese patients are at an increased risk for gallbladder disease and calculi formation. Answer 3 is incorrect as it is vital that the patient is alert for the onset of infection in order to facilitate early treatment. Answer 4 is the correct answer. The patient must be instructed to take this medication daily. Chenodeoxycholic acid (CDCA) is an agent that has been found to help dissolve or decrease the size of calculi in about 60 percent of patients with calculi of cholesterol materials. It works to prevent the formation of additional stones, as well, and should be taken daily.

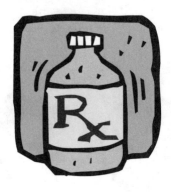

Questions

Diana suffers from recurrent bouts of cystitis. Upon presentation at this urgent visit, she tells you that she has had symptoms for about ten days including dysuria, frequency, and bladder area tenderness. Which of Diana's statements indicates that she may be suffering from an infection more complicated than cystitis?

1) "I have noticed some bright red blood in my urine."
2) "I have been experiencing some low back pain."
3) "I often feel as though I need to urinate but can't at times."
4) "I have been vomiting and have no desire to eat."

*Your Own Answer*_____

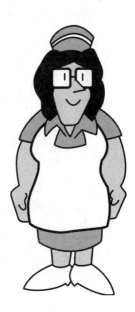

Correct Answers

This question deals with a chronic health problem which, as in this case, can lead to more serious illness if not promptly treated. Answer 1 is incorrect as hematuria is often present in uncomplicated cystitis. Mild low back pain may also be experienced making answer 2 incorrect. Bladder spasms due to irritation of the bladder lining may simulate the need to urinate and frequently is reported with cystitis, therefore, answer 3 is not the correct answer. Nausea, vomiting, and anorexia are important clues which may point to ascension of the infecting organism of a lower urinary through one or both ureters resulting in pyelonephritis, making answer 4 the correct answer to this question. Fever, chills, diarrhea, flank tenderness, and costa vertebral angle tenderness may be present as well.

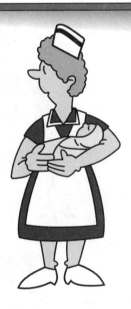

Questions

Q134

Billy has a history of seasonal allergic rhinitis usually managed by an antihistamine. From time to time he experiences minor nasal congestion and clear nasal discharge. Today, as you sign him in to the clinic and obtain a history, he states he feels as though he might have sinusitis. If this is the case you would expect him to report all of the following signs and symptoms EXCEPT:

1) thick nasal discharge that is dark green in color
2) persistent pain and pressure in and around his eyes
3) an aching in his upper teeth and gums
4) fever of 102°, shaking, chills, and vomiting

*Your Own Answer*_____

Q135

Eric is seen by the physician in the private office you are employed in. He is diagnosed via rapid culture with strep pharyngitis and placed on erythromycin for ten days. During patient teaching you tell him not to:

1) stop taking the antibiotic once his throat is no longer painful
2) gargle with warm water and salt to help reduce pain
3) be sure to drink plenty of water and other fluids
4) stay home from work while he is febrile and to get plenty of rest

*Your Own Answer*_____

Correct Answers

A134

Allergic rhinitis is a chronic condition due to local reaction of the nasal mucosa which may include swelling and the production of nasal discharge. An exacerbation of this process may cause the complication of sinusitis. This occurs when drainage is occluded by edema of the nasal mucosa and turbinates causing the growth of bacteria in the medium of excess mucous which infects the sinus cavities. Answer 1 is not the correct answer as this is often seen in sinusitis. Answer 2 is also incorrect as pressure and pain in this area may be attributed to infection/inflammation of the ethmoid sinuses. Answer 3 is not correct because maxillary sinusitis can sometimes mimic a toothache. Answer 4 is the correct answer. High fever with chills and vomiting are not common in sinusitis and may signal a serious complication (i.e., brain abscess in frontal sinusitis) or another disease process.

A135

This question focuses on avoiding serious medical complications from common illness such as strep pharyngitis through planning and implementation. Answer 1 is the correct answer to this question. Pharyngitis due to beta hemolytic step must be treated completely with a ten-day course of antibiotic. Incomplete cure may cause serious infection of the heart (endocarditis) or kidneys (glomerulonephritis). Answers 2, 3, and 4 are all incorrect as each statement consists of measures that will aid in the management and/or resolution of this acute illness.

Questions

Bob is a twenty-one-year-old patient with schizo-phrenia who is on several medications in an attempt to control taunting auditory hallucina-tions. No medications have been successful so far. Which action by the nurse may cause deteriora-tion in the patient while he is experiencing a period of increased symptoms?

1) gently reminding the patient that the voices that he's hearing are not real
2) consistently praising Bob when he responds positively to a stressor
3) arguing with the client when he insists "they keep yelling at me"
4) limiting background noise and extraneous en-vironmental stimuli

*Your Own Answer*_____

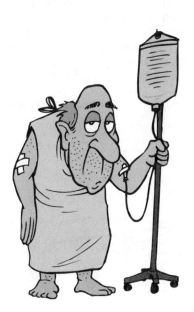

Correct Answers

Schizophrenia is theorized to occur from an inability to cope with the demands of reality. The patient becomes unable to interpret environmental cues correctly and often will enhance stimuli for the basis of their hallucinations, which are often frightening. Answer 1 is not the correct answer because reminding Bob that the voices are not real will assist him in adjusting his sensory perception toward a more realistic plane. Answer 2 is not the correct answer, either. Consistent positive reinforcement helps to imprint positive behaviors. Even small measures such as the patient taking a few deep breaths when he is frustrated should be acknowledged. Positive reinforcement also helps to increase self-esteem. Answer 3 is the correct answer as it illustrates an action which may cause escalation of the patient's discomfort and anxiety and potentiate violence. Patients with altered sensory perception should not be agitated or argued with to avoid an acute incident. The patient should be gently reassured that he is safe and that people are present to help him remain safe. Answer 4 is not the correct answer as it illustrates measures that will limit environmental stimuli and decrease the chance of the patient perceiving it incorrectly.

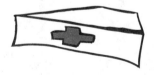

Questions

Travis is a twenty-three-year-old alcohol abuser mandated to an inpatient chemical dependency program. His pattern of abuse is that of episodic, compulsive indulgence in which he frequently becomes aggressive, violent, and experiences blackout periods during many of which he has gotten into legal trouble. Travis continues to deny that his problems are caused by his abuse of alcohol. Including which of the following in his care plan may be helpful:

1) allow Travis to miss those therapy meetings that he feels he doesn't need
2) confront Travis about his denial during a peer group therapy meeting
3) encourage long napping and rest periods throughout the day
4) identify a staff member to take responsibility for Travis' recovery

Your Own Answer

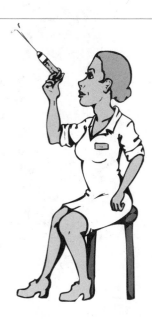

A137

This question deals with planning care for a patient with a chemical abuse problem. Answer 1 is incorrect. He should be encouraged to attend all therapy sessions so that he will listen to others who have experienced similar situations to his own. This may be thought provoking and encourage him to explore his situation. Answer 2 is correct because denial is easily identified by those who have had similar experiences. It may be helpful for him to hear perceptions of his situation by others. Answer 3 is incorrect as it allows the client to avoid confronting his denial and wastes time that could be spent working through the issues that underlay his problem. Answer 4 is also incorrect as only Travis can be held responsible for his own recovery.

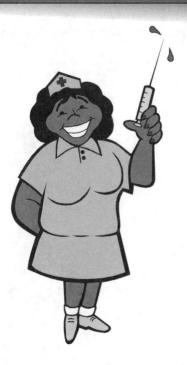

Questions

Joe is a recovering alcoholic. He has just been informed of the death of a friend and states that he is feeling the urge to have a drink. The nurse offers some suggestions which may be helpful to him. Which of the following is NOT:

1) allow yourself to experience the emotions that you are feeling even though they may be painful

2) share your feelings with a trusted person from a support group, your family, or your group of friends

3) keep your feelings to yourself so that you won't have to acknowledge that they are difficult to deal with

4) spend time thinking about your friend and of the foundation on which your relationship was based

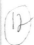

Your Own Answer_____

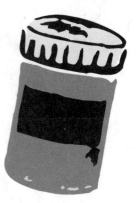

Correct Answers

Answer 3 is the correct answer to this question because it is the only suggestion that would NOT be helpful to Joe. Keeping his feelings to himself would keep him from getting the help he needs at this time. This question is based on assisting a person in recovery from chemical abuse to deal with stressors without self-medicating to blunt the difficult feelings. Answer 1 would be helpful to Joe because it recognizes that he is experiencing feelings that are difficult to deal with. Answer 2 is helpful to Joe because it encourages him to experience the pain of loss, keeps him in the present, and discourages his past use of alcohol for escaping pain. Answer 4 would help Joe because reflection can be insightful.

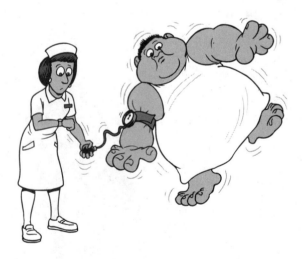

Questions

Q139

Mrs. Jones speaks to the nurse at the pediatrician's office about her 13-year-old daughter who has begun wearing garish makeup and unusual clothes. She has also cut her hair into a very severe, short, and unusual style. The nurse encourages Mrs. Jones not to worry and tells her that her daughter is:

1) trying to test the limits that her mother will allow her to reach with her hair, makeup, and clothes
2) trying to gain the attention of a certain peer group so that she will be able to fit in with the rest of them
3) exploring her personal identity and sense of self and style which is normal and important at her age
4) probably going to become a creative musician or abstract artist when she goes to college

*Your Own Answer*_____

Q140

Martha is an eighteen-year-old who has just returned from her first semester away at college. She talks incessantly about her new group of friends and has been dating one boy steadily for about two months. Martha seems to be successfully resolving her Eriksonian developmental tasks of which stage:

1) industry versus inferiority
2) integrity versus despair
3) trust versus mistrust
4) intimacy versus isolation

*Your Own Answer*_____

Correct Answers

This question deals with assisting patients and their families through the normal stages of growth and development. The nurse reassures the concerned parent in this question through implementing a plan to educate her on normal adolescent behaviors. Answer 1 is not the correct answer. Self-exploration is often confused with limit testing by uninformed parents. Answer 2 is incorrect although this behavior is seen during adolescence. Answer 3 is correct. Erikson identifies the adolescent period as confronting "identity versus role confusion." Answer 4 is incorrect. There is no evidence to support these assumptions.

This question deals with evaluating a patient's development throughout the lifespan. Answer 1 is incorrect as this task is accomplished during the school-age period of six to twelve years. Answer 2 is not the correct answer to this question. From approximately age sixty-five (or around retirement) until death, this developmental milestone is addressed. Answer 3 is incorrect, this task is resolved during infancy up until around the eighteenth month. Answer 4 is correct as this task is worked on from approximately age eighteen until twenty-five.

Questions

Q141

Mr. Adams has been diagnosed with terminal lung cancer and has a prognosis of approximately six months. He is seventy-five years old. Hospice care is arranged and the nurse and social worker work together to form a multidisciplinary approach to care. In planning some sessions for emotional support and counseling, both professionals agree that the patient should have assistance with which developmental task:

1) integrity versus despair
2) intimacy versus isolation
3) generativity versus stagnation
4) initiative versus guilt

*Your Own Answer*_____

Q142

Nancy is a wife and mother of three young adults who are all living at home. She knows that there is a strong family history of hypertension on both sides of the family. She is careful to serve well-balanced meals which are low in fat and in sodium content. Nancy's actions are an example of her:

1) desire to change her children's genetic predispositions
2) promotion of healthy habits to prevent the onset of disease
3) obsession with recipes from healthy living magazines
4) attempt to undo a lifetime of unhealthy eating habits

*Your Own Answer*_____

Correct Answers

A141

This question deals with planning of care to facilitate exploration and resolution of developmental tasks (as detailed by Erikson) for the dying patient. Answer 1 is the correct answer to this question. The dying patient should be assisted in exploring the tasks pertinent to his developmental stage. At this stage of life, especially after being diagnosed with a terminal disease, the manner in which one regards his life's accomplishments and failures is very important. Similarly important is the manner with which one accepts the certainty of death. Answer 2 is incorrect as this stage is addressed during young adulthood. Answer 3 is incorrect because this stage is dealt with during middle adulthood. Answer 4 is incorrect and concerns the late childhood period.

A142

This question deals with analysis of provided data. Answer 1 is incorrect because genetic traits are determined from conception and can't be changed. Answer 2 is the correct answer and is a good example of wellness promotion. Answer 3 is not the correct answer. This does not seem to be a negative hobby. Answer 4 is incorrect as it is never fruitless to adopt healthier habits.

Questions

Q143

Pulmonary tuberculosis is a disease which is easily communicable and can cause severe fibrosis and calcification within the lungs. In order to prevent spread of this disease and facilitate early diagnosis and treatment, which of the following should occur:

1) avoidance of contact with high risk patients
2) institution of mass screening using chest radiography
3) skin testing and treatment of those with active disease
4) prophylactic drug treatment for all at high risk

*Your Own Answer*_____

Q144

Influenza can cause a mild or serious to possibly fatal pneumonia in elderly or debilitated patients with chronic disease and some other high-risk groups. For this reason, all of the following should receive yearly influenza immunization EXCEPT:

1) persons with COPD
2) the diabetic patient
3) high school students
4) nursing home residents

*Your Own Answer*_____

Correct Answers

A143

This question discusses planning and implementation for disease prevention and early identification of tuberculosis (TB). Answer 1 is not the correct answer because this group encompasses many categories including the elderly, the debilitated and chronically ill, substance abusers, those who live in crowded areas, and those with poor nutrition and inadequate access to health care. Answer 2 is incorrect and an impractical and expensive means of screening. Answer 3 is the correct answer. A positive mantoux or purified protein derivative skin test for tuberculosis indicates either prior exposure to TB, active TB disease, or vaccination for TB (many foreign countries). Active disease is diagnosed by chest radiograph and clinical examination. Answer 4 is not the correct answer as this would not be an easy undertaking. TB requires combination drug therapy with drugs that potentiate many side effects.

A144

This question deals with prevention of disease and its complications and planning care for high risk groups. Answer 3 is the correct answer to this question as it identifies a group which does not require yearly influenza immunization, Answers 1, 2, and 4 are all incorrect answers. These groups all require yearly influenza immunization. It should also be noted that health care workers should receive yearly prophylactic influenza immunization.

Questions

Q145

Pneumococcal pneumonia, a bacterial pneumonia, can cause serious illness requiring hospitalization, intravenous antibiotics, and complications due to advanced age or chronic disease. Prevention of this illness is achieved via:

1) yearly influenza vaccination
2) administration of oral amantadine prophylaxis
3) proper rest and nutrition
4) a one-time immunization with pneumococcal vaccine

*Your Own Answer*_____

Q146

Mrs. Jones has been diagnosed with mitral valve prolapse with +2 mitral regurgitation. She has no other medical problems. In order to prevent the complication of infectious endocarditis, you remind Mrs. Jones to:

1) get an electrocardiogram and echocardiogram yearly
2) avoid participation in strenuous physical activity
3) limit dietary caffeine intake to no more than one cup daily
4) take prophylactic antibiotics when going to the dentist

*Your Own Answer*_____

Correct Answers

A145

This question looks at planning for prevention of potentially serious illness. Answer 1 is incorrect; influenza vaccination does not offer protection against pneumococcal pneumonia. Answer 2 is also incorrect. Amantadine is given to treat influenza within forty-eight hours of onset. Answer 3 may help to keep the immune system at its best, but, it is not the correct answer. Answer 4 is the correct answer to this question and is indicated for those over age sixty-five and with any chronic disease and possibly for those living in nursing residences.

A146

This question concerns health promotion and prevention of a serious potential complication due to a very common health problem, Answer 1 is not correct. These studies are obtained at time of diagnosis and depending on severity of the problem or signs and symptoms are redone periodically. Answer 2 is not the correct answer and this disease entity usually does not limit physical activity. Answer 3 is incorrect as caffeine consumption has no effect upon the contraction of endocarditis. Answer 4 is the correct answer to this question. It prevents bacteremic vegetation from attaching to the valve and causing endocarditis.

Questions

Q147

As the school nurse in a large high school, you realize the importance of your role in promoting health seeking behaviors. As you plan a series of awareness days on risk and injury prevention, you plan to cover all of the following topics except:

1) issues of sexuality, contraception, and sexually transmitted diseases
2) the risks of reckless driving and driving while impaired
3) problems relating to substance/chemical/alcohol abuse
4) how to get in to the college of your choice

*Your Own Answer*_____

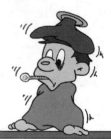

Q148

Jane, an eighteen-year-old female, is a patient in the diabetic clinic. You know she is taking an active roll in her care when she says:

1) "My fasting sugars are running slightly high."
2) "I'm sorry I missed the last appointment I had."
3) "I have my insulin, meter, and a snack with me."
4) "I woke up too late to test my sugar today."

*Your Own Answer*_____

Correct Answers

A147

This question deals with planning for health promotion in adolescence. Answers 1, 2, and 3 are incorrect as they are all important topics to discuss with this age group, which tends to see itself as immortal or invincible. This is evidenced by risk taking behaviors in all of these topics. Answer 4 is an important topic for teenagers but does not impact upon their health directly.

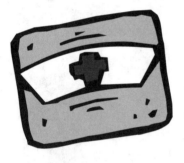

A148

This question evaluates the self-care behaviors of an adolescent client. Answer 1 is incorrect as it illustrates less than optimal glycemic control. Answer 2 is incorrect, another sign of irresponsibility, as is incorrect answer 4. Answer 3 indicates that Jane is prepared for her afternoon peak of NPH insulin with a snack and has her insulin and blood glucose meter in case she needs to adjust. These are all indicators of motivated self-care.

Questions

Q149

Ms. Andrews has been under many pressures at work and has been doing excessive amounts of typing to meet a deadline. She begins to develop pain in her wrists and some numbness in her fingers. You educate the patient to take which of the following measures for her carpal tunnel symptoms:

1) apply warm soaks, as ordered, to painful areas of the wrists
2) take Percocet, as prescribed, for severe pain in her wrists
3) begin her work on time so she won't need to rush for deadlines
4) ensure desk and keyboard are at anatomically correct angles

*Your Own Answer*_____

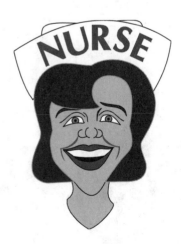

Correct Answers

A149

This question concerns self-care and health promotion. Answer 1 is not helpful in this disease process and is therefore incorrect. Cool compresses will often give relief of symptoms. Answer 2 is incorrect as an NSAID would probably lend more relief in this acute flair of symptoms. Answer 3 is not the correct answer but may be something for Jane to keep in mind to prevent further problems with her wrists. Answer 4 is the correct answer. An adjustment as simple as those suggested may alleviate symptoms by promoting typing in a more natural hand position.

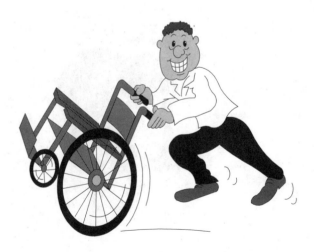

Questions

Ms. Bradford, a diabetic, is two days postoperative. On morning rounds, the nurse notices that she is sweating, but has cold and clammy skin, a pulse rate of 94/minute, and a BP reading of 80/50. The client says she is too weak to eat her breakfast and has asked repeatedly where she is and when she can return home. She is wringing her hands and tossing uncomfortably in the bed. The nurse's first actions would include the following:

1) help Ms. B. drink a glass of orange juice; she is having a hypoglycemic reaction
2) help Ms. B. drink a glass of orange juice; she is having a hyperglycemic reaction
3) remove the syrup from Ms. B.'s breakfast; she is having a hyperglycemic reaction
4) remove the syrup from Ms. B.'s breakfast; she is having a hypoglycemic reaction

*Your Own Answer*_____

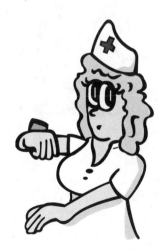

Correct Answers

Answer 1 is correct; these are the signs and symptoms of a hypoglycemic reaction. Therefore, answers 2 and 3 are incorrect. Answer 4 is also not the best choice; the nurse would want to administer, not remove, a food source of simple carbohydrates to this client in order to quickly raise her blood glucose level. Staying with the client while she finishes a glass of orange juice gives the nurse time to help calm and orient her as well as check her vital signs frequently until her pulse and BP return to normal.

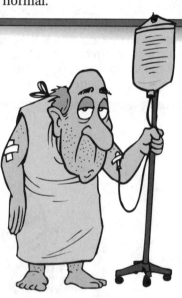

Questions

Q151

The nurse is meeting with a group of newly diagnosed clients with Type II (non-insulin dependent) diabetes. During a hypoglycemic event, an occurrence common in the management of diabetes, the nurse teaches the clients:

1) that strenuous exercise can greatly increase the blood sugar level
2) that carbohydrates and protein should be avoided before exercise
3) that food high in protein and fat and low in carbohydrates is best
4) that eating too much refined sugar decreases insulin secretion

*Your Own Answer*_____

Q152

Chronic hyperglycemia is best characterized by:

1) weight gain, excessive hunger, decreased urination, and excessive thirst
2) weight gain, anorexia, increased urination, and decreased thirst
3) weight loss, anorexia, decreased urination, and excessive thirst
4) weight loss, excessive hunger, excessive urination, and excessive thirst

*Your Own Answer*_____

Correct Answers

A151

Answer 3 is correct. A diet high in protein and fat, and especially devoid of simple carbohydrates, is recommended for the hypoglycemic client. Strenuous exercise serves to lower blood sugar levels, and so complex carbohydrates and protein—which convert most easily to a usable form of energy—should be eaten just before and/or after exercise. A diet high in refined sugar tends to stimulate insulin secretion. Therefore, answers 1, 2, and 4 are incorrect.

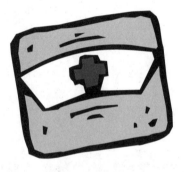

A152

Answer 4 is correct. Polyphagia (excessive hunger), polyuria (excessive urination), polydypsia (excessive thirst), and weight loss accompany the hyperglycemia which, along with these symptoms, is diagnostic of diabetes.

Questions

Q153

In taking a 30-year-old female client's personal and family medical history during her annual checkup, the nurse elicits the following information: the client's mother and maternal grandmother died of breast and colon cancer, respectively, and her father and brother have diabetes; she has been overweight or obese for much of her life, as she is currently; she had an appendectomy at age 7 and pneumonia at age 12; she has a son and a daughter, both born full-term, weighing 10.5 and 11 pounds, respectively; and she and her husband are planning to have a third child in the next year. The nurse will expect to draw bloods for the following lab values:

1) chemistry, hematology, liver function tests, and an STD panel
2) chemistry, hematology, thyroid function tests, and a 3-hour GTT
3) chemistry, hematology, blood urea nitrogen, and an HIV test
4) chemistry, hematology, creatinine clearance test, and a viral survey

*Your Own Answer*_____

Q154

The nurse is aware that an oral or IV glucose tolerance test would not generally be performed on:

1) an obese person
2) a pregnant woman
3) a known diabetic
4) a cancer survivor

*Your Own Answer*_____

Correct Answers

A153

Answer 2 is the best choice. The nurse would expect the standard labs to be ordered, along with a 3-hour glucose tolerance test on a client with a family history of diabetes, a history of obesity, and two full-term babies each born weighing more than 10 pounds. Tests for most STDs are not done through bloodwork; an HIV test would be done at the request of the client; and a creatinine clearance test is done on urine, not blood.

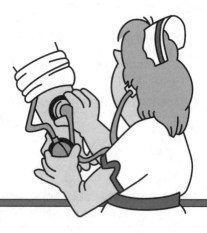

A154

Answer 3 is correct. Seventy-five grams of glucose solution are administered in a bolus dose which, in a known diabetic, could cause a severe hyperglycemic reaction.

Questions

The priority nursing goal in the educa
newly-diagnosed diabetic clients is to te
clients to maintain control over their plas:
cose levels by:

1) controlling food portions
2) obtaining regular exercise
3) slow, gradual weight loss
4) all of the above

*Your Own Answer*_____

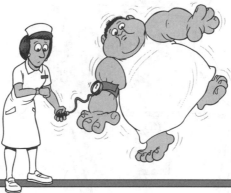

Q156

The nurse knows that it is important to assess the preoperative client for fluid and electrolyte balance, one component of which is fluid volume. This can be done indirectly through which measure(s)?

1) auscultating lung sounds
2) measurement of daily weight
3) assessment of skin turgor
4) all of the above

*Your Own Answer*_____

A155

Answer 4 is correct; all three management strategies are important to controlling diabetes and postponing the progression of complications.

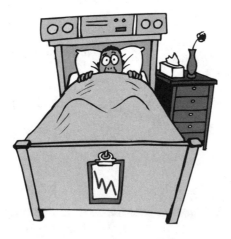

A156

Answer 4 is correct. These are all methods of indirect fluid volume evaluation, information that is valuable preoperatively to assess readiness for surgery as well as risks for postoperative complications.

Questions

Pulse rate, taken as a serial reading, can give the nurse information about fluid volume and electrolyte balance, among other things. The nurse should palpate the radial pulse:

1) for at least 30 seconds to determine rate, regularity, and volume
2) for at least 2 minutes to determine if there is a heart murmur
3) for no more than 15 seconds to determine rate and regularity only
4) for at least 30 seconds to determine rate and heart sounds

Your Own Answer⎯⎯⎯⎯⎯⎯⎯⎯⎯⎯⎯⎯⎯⎯⎯⎯⎯⎯⎯

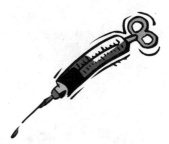

Q158

The type of lung sounds heard with fluid volume overload are:

1) wheezing on inspiration only
2) wheezing on expiration only
3) rales that don't clear with coughing
4) rhonchi bilaterally on inspiration

Your Own Answer⎯⎯⎯⎯⎯⎯⎯⎯⎯⎯⎯⎯⎯⎯⎯⎯⎯⎯⎯

Correct Answers

A157

Answer 1 is correct. The radial pulse should be assessed for at least 30 seconds, with this number then doubled to determine beats per minute. Assessment of volume is important in distinguishing between a bounding vs. thready pulse. Heart sounds, including extra sounds like a murmur, can only be discerned by auscultation at the apical pulse in the area of the heart. Therefore, answers 2, 3, and 4 are incorrect.

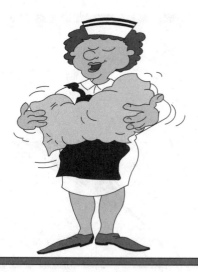

A158

Answer 3 is correct. As pulmonary congestion due to fluid volume overload increases, rales progress from the lower to the upper areas of the lungs. Wheezing is usually a result of bronchial obstruction. "Rhonchi" is often used interchangeably with "wheezing."

Questions

Q159

The most important factor determining how well a client might tolerate anesthesia and surgery is:

1) gastrointestinal system function
2) age and weight
3) financial resources
4) cardiopulmonary function

*Your Own Answer*_____

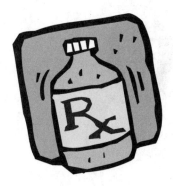

Q160

Mr. Samuels, an elderly client, has just arrived on the med-surg floor after undergoing GI surgery. The nurse knows it is important to assess him for fluid volume deficit. The first indication is usually:

1) decreased intake and output
2) orthostatic hypotension
3) confusion and restlessness
4) elevated blood pressure and pulse

*Your Own Answer*_____

Correct Answers

A159

The correct answer is 4. Adequate blood supply, a heart that pumps efficiently, blood vessel function, and efficient gas exchange are all important in decreasing the risk of complications peri- and postoperatively.

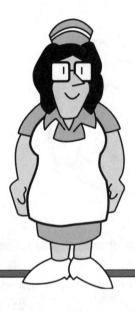

A160

Answer 2 is correct. Elevated BP and pulse might be early signs of fluid volume overload. Decreased I and O, confusion, and restlessness might be later indications of fluid volume deficit. Therefore, answers 1, 3, and 4 are not the best choices.

Questions

Q161

At 9:00 AM the nurse notices that an elderly client has not touched her breakfast, and is complaining of nausea, fatigue, and muscle weakness. On further assessment, the nurse notes abdominal distention and mild heart dysrhythmias. The client also reports that she has not had a bowel movement for the past 48 hours. The nurse calls the physician, suspecting which electrolyte imbalance:

1) hypernatremia
2) hyponatremia
3) hyperkalemia
4) hypokalemia

*Your Own Answer*_____

Q162

In order to assess the client for right-sided congestive heart failure, the nurse will prepare him for which procedure:

1) intra-aortic balloon pump
2) central venous pressure monitoring
3) percutaneous transluminal coronary angioplasty
4) pulmonary artery pressure monitoring

*Your Own Answer*_____

Correct Answers

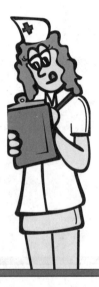

A161

Answer 4 is correct; these are presenting signs and symptoms of decreased serum potassium. With hyperkalemia and hyponatremia, diarrhea and abdominal cramps, but not distention, would be present. Hypernatremia would present with dry, sticky mucous membranes and nervousness.

A162

Answer 2 is the correct choice. A catheter is inserted into the superior vena cava or into the right atrium to assess function. Pulmonary artery monitoring is used to assess ventricular function. PTCA is used for the treatment of CAD and to assess for MI. An intraortic balloon pump is used in the treatment of cardiogenic shock.

Questions

Q163

One possible sign of elevated venous pressure in the client with excess fluid volume or congestive heart failure is:

1) jugular venous distention > 2 cm above the sternal angle when the client is sitting at a 45-degree angle
2) jugular venous distention > 4 cm above the sternal angle when the client is sitting at a 60-degree angle
3) subclavian venous distention > 2 cm above the sternal angle when the client is lying supine
4) subclavian venous distention > 4 cm above the sternal angle when the client is sitting at a 45-degree angle

*Your Own Answer*_____

Q164

Preoperative preparation of your client with COPD who is scheduled for abdominal surgery always includes which of the following actions:

1) IV fluid therapy, smoking cessation, and deep breathing exercises 1 month prior to surgery
2) daily measurement of fluid Intake and Output, and oxygen therapy at least 1 week prior to surgery
3) administration of bronchodilators, smoking cessation, and chest PT 1 week prior to surgery
4) aerobic exercise, daily measurement of Intake and Output, and vitamin therapy 1 week prior to surgery

*Your Own Answer*_____

Correct Answers

Answer 1 is correct. Normally when a client is lying supine, the jugular veins, located bilaterally on the anterior-lateral sides of the neck, fill to the anterior border of the SCM muscle. With the head raised to a 45-degree angle, the jugular venous pulsations should not be visible above the measurement of 2-3 cm from the sternal angle. Therefore, answer 2 is incorrect. Subclavian venous pressure is not used as an indicator of compromised cardiac function; therefore, answers 3 and 4 are incorrect.

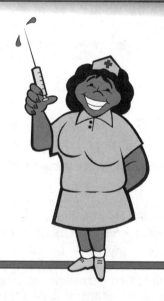

Answer 3 is the best choice. These three interventions decrease the likelihood of pulmonary complications postoperatively in the client with compromised pulmonary function at the outset.

Questions

Q165

In preparing a client for surgery, the nurse takes a medical history, performs a physical assessment, and evaluates lab results. Findings include a history of urinary frequency and nocturia, ankle edema, slightly elevated blood pressure, and proteinuria/hypoalbuminemia. The nurse's first action is to:

1) admit this client to the ER, with a suspicion of renal failure
2) call the physician; this client needs further evaluation
3) prepare this client for hemodialysis treatment instead of surgery
4) cancel the surgery; this client could not withstand the stress

*Your Own Answer*_____

Q166

The nurse's preoperative client is an insulin-dependent diabetic. The day before surgery, the nurse realizes that there is no order for insulin in the client's chart. The nurse should:

1) assume the client does not need to take the medication since she'll be NPO after midnight anyway
2) ask the client what amount of insulin she usually takes and give it according to the client's usual schedule
3) contact the physician to have an order written for insulin and administer it accordingly
4) mention this omission to the surgeon and anesthesiologist in the OR on the day of surgery

*Your Own Answer*_____

Correct Answers

A165

Answer 2 is the best choice. Surgery is not necessarily contraindicated in a client with potential renal disease, due to improved surgical management techniques. While these symptoms alone do not indicate renal failure, compromised renal function can progress to renal failure postoperatively. Therefore, this client requires further evaluation by the physician.

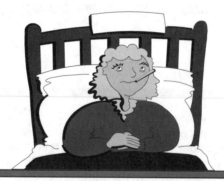

A166

Answer 3 is the best answer. Regular medications should be taken according to the dose and schedule the client's physician wishes to maintain throughout the perioperative period. Because an order does not exist in a client's chart, it may mean that the physician forgot to write it. It is the nurse's responsibility to elicit from the client a complete list of medications regularly taken, including aspirin, vitamins, etc.

Questions

Q167

Which of the following is placed in a biohazard "red" bag:

1) a blood-stained cotton hospital gown
2) blood-covered latex gloves
3) a needle used for an IM injection
4) each of the above

Your Own Answer

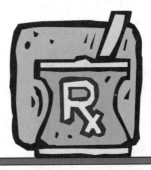

Q168

Ms. Richards has been admitted to the medical surgical unit 24 hours prior to a scheduled liver biopsy and possible exploratory surgery. In taking a preoperative history, the nurse has skillfully elicited the client's continuing alcohol abuse. While hospitalized, the client will most likely experience:

1) constipation, diarrhea, or other GI-system problems postoperatively
2) gratitude for the opportunity to stop drinking during hospitalization
3) an increased tolerance for the stress of surgery and anesthesia
4) alcohol withdrawal, with increased risk for infection postoperatively

Your Own Answer

Correct Answers

A167

Answer 2 is correct. The nondisposable soiled hospital gown belongs in a dirty-linens bag, where it will be properly cleaned by the hospital laundry service. Therefore, answer 1 is not the best choice. The used needle must be disposed of in a sharps container, which has an opening too small to put one's hands into and which will only be opened by personnel trained in safe disposal. Answers 3 and 4 are therefore incorrect.

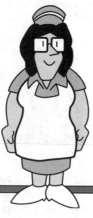

A168

Answer 4 is the correct choice. Alcohol withdrawal includes delirium tremens (which increase metabolic rate) and impaired immune response to infection, with a 50 percent increase in postoperative mortality rates. Chronic alcoholism diminishes the tolerance for stress due to decreased adrenocortical response. Postoperative GI symptoms are not exclusive to the chronic alcoholic. The client will probably express anger and hostility during the withdrawal period, which should be completed before surgery is performed.

Questions

Q169

The nurse knows it is important to question a pre-operative client about any known food, drug, or environmental allergies. When the client reports that she is allergic to iodine, the nurse's best line of questioning is:

1) "Is everyone in your family allergic to iodine? Do they have any other allergies?"
2) "Are there any other foods or drugs you are allergic to? Which ones might those be?"
3) "Have you ever experienced side effects from drugs? What about environmental allergies?"
4) "When did the reaction to iodine occur? How long did it last? What stopped the reaction?"

*Your Own Answer*_____

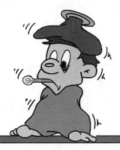

Q170

Adequate hematologic function is important to positive surgical and postoperative outcomes. Which of the following is an absolute contraindication to surgery:

1) pneumonia
2) history of smoking
3) use of aspirin
4) mild anemia

*Your Own Answer*_____

Correct Answers

A169

Answer 4 is the best choice. To some clients, an allergic reaction can mean fatal anaphylactic shock. It is important to elicit details regarding the allergic response the client has mentioned before going on to complete the client's personal and family allergy history.

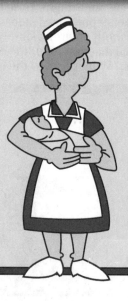

A170

Answer 1 is correct. Pneumonia must be resolved before surgery can be performed due to the accompanying impairment of respiratory function. Smoking, regular use of aspirin, and mild anemia may increase the risk of postoperative hemorrhage, but if managed properly are not absolute contraindications. Therefore, answers 2, 3, and 4 are not the best choices.

 Take Test-Readiness Quiz 2 on CD
(to review questions 87–170)

Questions

Q171

The nurse caring for an 80-year-old postoperative client knows that her age increases the likelihood of development of sequelae. Which of the following is least likely to occur:

1) hypoxemia and shock
2) venous thrombosis
3) pressure sores
4) orthostatic hypotension

*Your Own Answer*_____

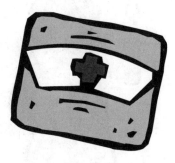

Q172

Common nursing diagnoses for the preoperative client are least likely to include:

1) knowledge deficit related to surgical procedure
2) depression related to possible surgical findings
3) ineffective coping strategies related to upcoming surgery
4) alteration in nutritional status: less than body requirement

*Your Own Answer*_____

Correct Answers

A171

Answer 3 is correct. All except pressure sores, which are an integumentary system complication, are possible postoperative cardiovascular sequelae for which the elderly postoperative client in particular is at risk. Therefore, answers 1, 2, and 4 are not the best choices.

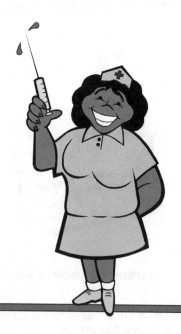

A172

Answer 2 is the best choice. This is a psychiatric diagnosis, while all the rest—answers 1, 3, and 4—are nursing diagnoses to be expected with a preoperative client.

Questions

Q173

An incentive spirometer is used by the postoperative client in order to:

1) produce increased lung volume
2) enhance venous return
3) help the client take slow, deep breaths
4) all of the above

*Your Own Answer*_____

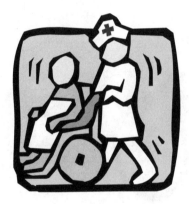

Q174

The nurse teaches the postoperative client not to use an incentive spirometer immediately before or after meals because it may cause:

1) nausea
2) a hypotensive crisis
3) a hypertensive crisis
4) abdominal distention

*Your Own Answer*_____

Correct Answers

A173

Answer 4 is correct. These are the goals for the postoperative client utilizing the incentive spirometer in order to avoid respiratory complications.

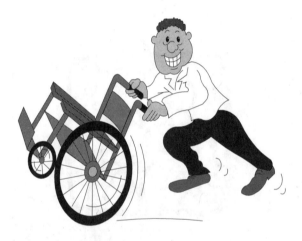

A174

Answer 1 is correct. For the comfort of the client, it is best to time incentive spirometer use for times between meals. Abdominal distention or severe changes in blood pressure are not likely to occur as a result of using an incentive spirometer immediately before or after meals. Therefore, answers 2, 3, and 4 are not the best choices.

Questions

Q175

The best time for the postoperative client to use the incentive spirometer is:

1) immediately before breakfast, lunch, and dinner
2) immediately after breakfast, lunch, and dinner
3) immediately before and after voiding urine
4) anytime other than immediately before or after meals

*Your Own Answer*_____

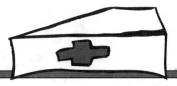

Q176

The best position for the postoperative client to maintain during deep-breathing exercises is:

1) prone
2) semi-Fowler's
3) supine
4) forward-leaning

*Your Own Answer*_____

Correct Answers

A175

Answer 4 is correct. In order to avoid nausea, it is best not to use the incentive spirometer immediately before or after meals. Answers 1, 2, and 3 are not the best choices.

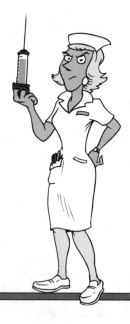

A176

Answer 2 is the best choice. Deep breathing postoperatively promotes the reinflation of alveoli in the lungs, as well as the even distribution of surfactant, in order to keep them from collapsing. The other 3 positions, answers 1, 3, and 4, are not as conducive to ease of deep-breathing due to pressure exerted on the diaphragm.

Questions

Q177

The nurse teaches the client with an abdominal or upper-thoracic incision to cough without creating too much tension on the wound by which of the following technique(s):

1) stick out the tongue when coughing
2) splint the incision with a pillow when coughing
3) both answers 1 and 2
4) neither answers 1 nor 2

*Your Own Answer*_____

Q178

Postoperative pulmonary complications can be best prevented by all of the following interventions except:

1) helping the client turn from side to side at least every 2 hours
2) assisting the client to a modified sitting position
3) keeping the client comfortable and non-ambulatory
4) performing passive range-of-motion leg exercises

*Your Own Answer*_____

Correct Answers

A177

Answer 3 is correct. These are both effective techniques for splinting the wound when coughing. With less pain, the client is more likely to cough often enough to lower the risk of postoperative respiratory complications.

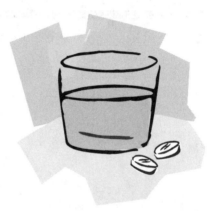

A178

Answer 3 is correct. Helping the client turn from side to side helps loosen lung secretions. In a modified sitting position, perfusion and ventilation are improved in the lungs. Passive ROM as well as the client actively exercising leg muscles will prepare him or her for early ambulation. While the client should be kept as comfortable and pain-free as possible, early ambulation must be encouraged and assisted, unless contraindicated by the surgery itself.

Questions

Q179

The nurse instructs postoperative clients to ask for pain medication:

1) on a predetermined regular schedule
2) when the pain becomes very severe
3) before the pain becomes very severe
4) preferably once during each nursing shift

Your Own Answer

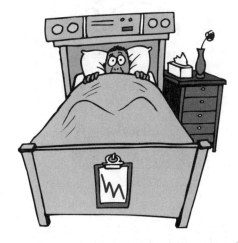

Q180

According to research regarding postoperative pain medication, nurses tend to:

1) overmedicate
2) undermedicate
3) medicate appropriately
4) forget to medicate

Your Own Answer

Correct Answers

A179

Answer 3 is the best choice. The client should learn to intercept pain by asking for medication before the pain is unendurable. A predetermined regular schedule will not allow for the interception of pain. Therefore, answers 1 and 4 are not good choices. Once the pain becomes severe (answer 2), a greater than usual amount of medication is necessary to achieve relief.

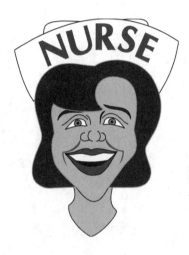

A180

Answer 2 is correct. This may be due to a fear of the client becoming psychologically or physically dependent on the pain medication, especially if it is a narcotic. Therefore, answers 1, 3, and 4 are not correct.

Questions

Q181

The nurse teaches the preoperative client that she should not eat for 8 to 12 hours prior to the time of the scheduled surgery. The client demonstrates her understanding of this instruction when she says:

1) "I am to have nothing by mouth—neither food nor water—for 8 to 12 hours before surgery in order to avoid throwing up during surgery."
2) "I am to have nothing by mouth—neither food nor water—for 8 to 12 hours before surgery in order to avoid abdominal bloating during surgery."
3) "I am to have nothing by mouth—neither food nor water—for 8 to 12 hours before surgery in order to avoid having to urinate during surgery."
4) "I am to eat no solid food at all 8 to 12 hours before surgery, but drinking coffee, tea, milk, or fruit juice is not a problem."

*Your Own Answer*_____

Q182

The nurse is aware that the client who was malnourished preoperatively will most often suffer which postoperative complication:

1) poor wound healing
2) ulcerative decubiti
3) hypoxemia and shock
4) pulmonary infection

*Your Own Answer*_____

Correct Answers

A181

Answer 1 is the best choice. Vomiting during surgery can lead to aspiration, which in turn can lead to pneumonia, with a 50 percent-90 percent mortality rate, depending on the amount of gastric contents aspirated. Abdominal bloating perioperatively is not usually life-threatening; answer 2 is therefore not the best choice. While under general anesthesia, urine is collected in a pouch via a urinary catheter inserted in the urethra; therefore, answer 3 is incorrect. Ingesting liquids as well as solids preoperatively can cause vomiting and aspiration. Therefore, answer 4 is not a good choice.

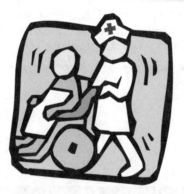

A182

Answer 1 is the correct choice. Good wound healing is enhanced by a balanced diet, with high carbohydrate and especially high protein content. Answers 2, 3, and 4 are not generally the expected postoperative complications in the preoperatively malnourished client.

Questions

Q183

Total parenteral nutrition (TPN) is often used pre-operatively to correct or reduce protein deficiency and to avoid the postoperative complications of hypoproteinemia. Which of the following nursing goals may be met through the use of TPN:

1) reduction of edema at the wound site
2) increase in resistance to infection
3) acceleration of wound healing
4) all of the above

*Your Own Answer*_____

Q184

The nurse knows to ask the preoperative client to remove her nail polish and makeup before surgery because:

1) they make it difficult to assess the nailbeds and skin perioperatively
2) there is greater likelihood of an allergic reaction to the anesthesia
3) they are distracting to the operating room staff and to the surgeon
4) they are unhygienic and could lead to postoperative infection

*Your Own Answer*_____

Correct Answers

A183

Answer 4 is correct. Protein supplementation, obtained through TPN, can meet all of these post-operative nursing goals.

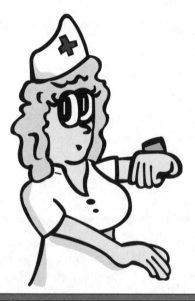

A184

Answer 1 is correct. Skin color and nailbeds must be observed perioperatively to assess the client for hypoxemia and poor circulation.

Questions

Q185

Which of the following items would not be removed prior to surgery:

1) a wig
2) jewelry
3) a hearing aid
4) dentures

*Your Own Answer*_____

Q186

The usual dose of preoperative medication for an elderly client is generally:

1) reduced compared to a younger client
2) increased compared to a younger client
3) the same as that for a younger client
4) related to factors other than age

*Your Own Answer*_____

Q187

Preoperative or preanesthesia medications are used in order to:

1) create amnesia for the preoperative events
2) minimize the client's anxiety
3) decrease the needed amount of anesthesia
4) all of the above

*Your Own Answer*_____

Correct Answers

A185

Answer 3 is the best choice. The nurse must inform the OR staff that the client has a hearing aid in place. Answer 1 is incorrect; however, if the client does not wish to be seen without a wig, it can be removed after anesthesia is given. Answer 2 is incorrect because, other than a plain wedding band that can be taped to the client's finger, all jewelry must be removed prior to surgery. Answer 4 is also incorrect because dentures can slip out of place and block the pharynx during anesthesia.

A186

Answer 1 is the best choice. Severe respiratory depression can ensue with use of opioid analgesics, the most commonly prescribed preoperative medication. Therefore, some anesthesiologists prefer to prescribe only benzodiazepines or mild sedatives to elderly clients. Answers 2, 3, and 4 are not the best choices.

A187

Answer 4 is correct. All of these are the desired effects of preoperative medication.

Questions

Q188

Once the nurse has administered the preoperative medication to the client, the next priority intervention would be to:

1) arrange for a loved one to be at the surgical client's bedside
2) raise the siderails of the bed and give the client the call button
3) arrange for the client's postoperative meals by phoning the kitchen
4) arrange for transport of the client to the holding area of the OR

*Your Own Answer*_____

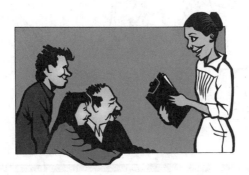

Q189

The surgical client is most likely to acquire an infection:

1) from the hospital's food
2) from his or her roommate
3) while in the operating room
4) upon returning home

*Your Own Answer*_____

Correct Answers

A188

Answer 2 is the best choice. The nurse will also instruct the client to remain in bed once medicated. All the other actions would occur once the client's safety had been ensured.

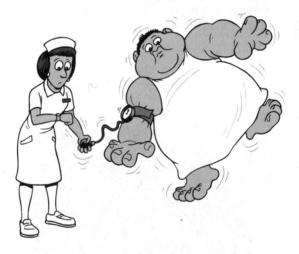

A189

Answer 3 is correct. Nosocomial, or hospital-acquired, infections, especially while in the OR, are more common than any other in the perioperative client. Therefore, answers 1, 2, and 4 are not the best choices. Appropriate hair removal and skin preparation prior to surgery minimize the risk of acquiring a wound infection while in the OR.

Questions

Q190

The purpose of draping a surgical client is to:
1) establish a sterile field around the operative site
2) protect the client's privacy and sense of modesty
3) create psychological distance for the surgeon
4) keep the scrub nurse from witnessing the surgery

Your Own Answer

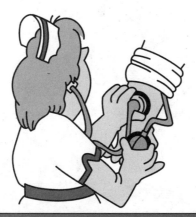

Q191

Which one of the following is the least important reason for wound drainage?

1) puts pressure on surrounding organs
2) is a medium for bacteria
3) may cause a hypertensive crisis
4) may prevent proper wound closure

Your Own Answer

Correct Answers

A190

Answer 1 is correct. The sterile field will help prevent microorganisms from passing between sterile and nonsterile areas. While answers 2 and 3 have some validity, they are not the main purpose for draping a surgical client. Answer 4 is incorrect; the scrub nurse should not be kept from being aware of the progress of the surgery.

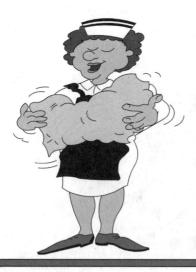

A191

Answer 3 is the correct choice. All of the other choices are reasons for the importance of draining a wound that is expected to accumulate large amounts of fluid.

Questions

The nurse's plan of care for a postoperative client with an abdominal incision dressing includes which of the following goals:

1) to protect the incision from microorganisms and trauma
2) to minimize edema at the incision and surrounding areas
3) to promote the client's esthetic and psychological comfort
4) each of the above

*Your Own Answer*_____

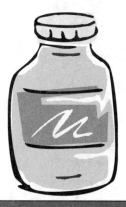

Q193

The nurse is aware that, when changing a wound dressing, the old dressing must be checked for:

1) amount of drainage
2) color of the drainage
3) odor of the drainage
4) all of the above

*Your Own Answer*_____

Correct Answers

A192

Answer 4 is the best choice. Each of these would be an objective for the nurse caring for a client with a wound dressing.

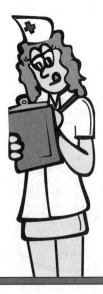

A193

Answer 4 is correct. The nurse assesses the wound dressing for each of these factors and documents this information in the client's chart. The physician or surgeon must be notified if signs of infection are noted by the nurse.

Questions

Q194

The nurse with a postoperative day 4 surgical client is changing the client's wound dressing when it is noted that the wound is malodorous and draining copious amounts of pus. The nurse's first intervention would be to:

1) take a wound culture and send it to the lab, and administer IV antibiotics
2) insert a wound drain at the incisional site and begin closed wound drainage
3) re-dress the wound, using strict asepsis, and notify the physician immediately
4) prepare the client for immediate surgery and repair of the wound

*Your Own Answer*_____

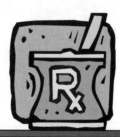

Q195

The time of recovery from general anesthesia is:

1) shorter than the time for induction
2) equal to the time for induction
3) longer than the time for induction
4) dependent on the ethnicity of the client

*Your Own Answer*_____

Correct Answers

A194

Answer 3 is the nurse's best choice. A wound culture and IV antibiotics would be administered on the order of the physician. A drain would not be inserted into the original incision, but rather through a nearby incision, usually created at the time of the original surgery. Immediate surgery and wound repair would be ordered in the case of wound evisceration.

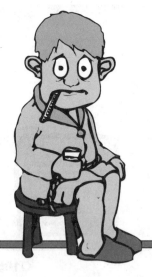

A195

Answer 3 is correct. Upon induction, the anesthesia moves quickly from the bloodstream to the tissues. During maintenance, fatty tissue stores the medication, and then gives it up more slowly due to its sparse blood supply. Therefore, answers 1, 2, and 4 are incorrect.

Questions

Q196

Reorder the following to show the order of recovery of reflexes from general anesthesia:

A) drowsiness
B) awake but disoriented
C) unconsciousness
D) response to stimuli

*Your Own Answer*_____

Q197

Immediate postoperative assessment by the recovery room nurse is least likely to include:

1) auscultating all lobes of the lungs
2) evaluating the level of consciousness
3) immediately initiating oxygen therapy
4) evaluating mucous membrane color

*Your Own Answer*_____

Q198

After transporting the immediate postoperative client to the recovery room, the nurse's single most important assessment is for:

1) tissue perfusion
2) airway patency
3) GI function
4) psychological state

*Your Own Answer*_____

Correct Answers

A196

C, D, B, A gives the correct order for the return of reflexes, which occurs in the reverse order in which they disappeared.

A197

Answer 3 is the correct choice. All three other choices are essential to the evaluation of respiratory function in the immediate postoperative client. Although the initiation of oxygen therapy is performed for all postoperative clients as soon as they enter the recovery room, this choice does not represent an assessment measure.

A198

Answer 2 is the best choice. The postoperative client's immediate well-being is primarily dependent on adequate ventilation. Postanesthesia complications often involve respiratory depression. The other choices, answers 1, 3, and 4, are important assessments after adequate ventilation has been established.

Questions

Q199

The first of the senses that returns to the client who has been under general anesthesia is:

1) hearing
2) smell
3) sight
4) touch

*Your Own Answer*_____

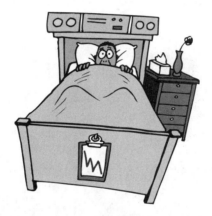

Q200

The nurse is aware of the importance of assessing for respiratory distress in the immediate postoperative client who received general anesthesia. Which of the following is the <u>least</u> reliable early sign of respiratory distress:

1) cyanosis
2) rapid, thready pulse
3) flaring nares
4) intercostal retractions

*Your Own Answer*_____

Correct Answers

A199

Answer 1 is correct. The recovery room nurse should speak to the client at normal volume and inform the client beforehand of when a procedure or an assessment will be performed. Smell, clear vision, and touch are all later to return postanesthesia. Therefore, answers 2, 3, and 4 are not the best choices.

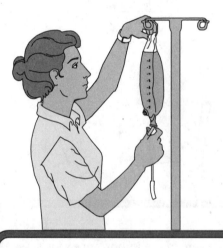

A200

Answer 1 is correct. Cyanosis is a later sign of respiratory distress, and is often unreliable due to variations in lighting and room temperature. Rapid, thready pulse and flaring nares with visible intercostal retractions—answers 2, 3, and 4—are all reliable signs of respiratory difficulty in any situation.

Questions

Q201

At the 15-minute vital signs assessment, the recovery room nurse notes that a postoperative client who returned from surgery half an hour ago has a blood pressure reading of 90/60, compared to her baseline measurements of 130/75 and 125/70. The nurse's priority intervention is:

1) to contact the surgeon and anesthesiologist and prepare the client to return to the operating room
2) to increase by double the client's intravenous fluids to avoid the onset of hypovolemic shock
3) to obtain arterial blood gas and chem-20 samples, suspecting an electrolyte imbalance
4) to continue to monitor vital signs q 15 minutes; slight hypotension is normal in healthy postop clients

*Your Own Answer*_____

Q202

The nurse is aware that the client who has been intubated prior to surgery will not be extubated until:

1) reflexes controlling coughing and swallowing return
2) client is awake enough to request the tubing be removed
3) client has received at least 3 hours of oxygen therapy
4) nurse notes the return to normal of all vital signs

*Your Own Answer*_____

Correct Answers

A201

Answer 4 is the best choice. Anesthetic agents may cause slight hypotension through peripheral vasodilation. This slight drop in blood pressure is generally well tolerated and need not be treated. Therefore, answers 1, 2, and 3 are not the best choices.

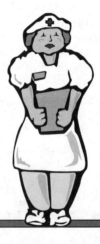

A202

Answer 1 is correct. The artificial airway is removed when the patient regains consciousness and is able to maintain his/her own airway. An oropharyngeal tube is removed when the client begins to swallow, or if he/she gags on the tubing, but not usually at the client's request, as in incorrect answer 2. The amount of O_2 therapy and the return to normal of vital signs, while important, are not determinants of the appropriate time to extubate a patient. Therefore answers 3 and 4 are not good choices.

Questions

Q203

The recovery room nurse notes that for a client with COPD there is an order for postoperative administration of 60 percent humid oxygen at a flow rate of 9 L. The nurse's plan of care for this client includes:

1) administering the oxygen as ordered by the physician
2) administering 80 percent oxygen at a rate of flow of 12 L
3) questioning the physician's order for this percentage of O2
4) questioning the physician's order for this rate of flow of O2

*Your Own Answer*_____

Q204

The primary purpose of deep-breathing, sighing, and yawning postoperatively is:

1) prevention of respiratory infection
2) prevention of bilateral atelectasis
3) return of facial muscle movement
4) relaxation for management of pain

*Your Own Answer*_____

Correct Answers

A203

Answer 3 is the best choice. Clients with COPD would receive a lower percentage of O2 than usual because the stimulus to breathe is a decrease in blood O2 level. Their respiratory drive would be obliterated by the administration of a high concentration of oxygen. Therefore answers 1 and 2 are incorrect. Answer 4 is also not a good choice, as the rate of flow is acceptable for this client.

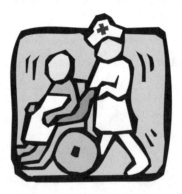

A204

Answer 2 is correct. These techniques help maintain the normal residual capacity of the lungs through the hyperinflation of the alveoli, resulting in the reversal of temporary atelectasis caused by inhalation anesthetics. Answer 1 is incorrect: these maneuvers will not necessarily prevent infection. Answers 3 and 4 might be secondary benefits of these techniques.

Questions

Q205

Mr. Dunn was scheduled for a tracheostomy after experiencing a stroke. The nurse includes in her plan of care for this client hyperventilation with:

1) 60 percent oxygen before beginning the suctioning process
2) 100 percent oxygen after finishing the suctioning process
3) 60 percent oxygen after each insertion of the suctioning catheter
4) 100 percent oxygen before the start of suctioning and then after each insertion of the suctioning catheter

*Your Own Answer*_____

Q206

Naloxone is sometimes used postoperatively as a narcotic antagonist for the reversal of respiratory depression from opiate narcotics. However, naloxone also:

1) is always highly psychologically addictive
2) usually induces vomiting and aspiration
3) interrupts the analgesic effect of opiates
4) causes bradycardia and hypotension

*Your Own Answer*_____

Correct Answers

A205

Answer 4 is the best choice. The oxygen that is removed during the suctioning process must be replaced each time with 100 percent oxygen before suctioning can be repeated, and again when the process is completed. Therefore, answers 1, 2, and 3 are not the best choices.

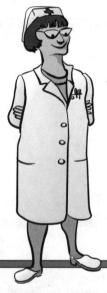

A206

Answer 3 is correct. Intense postoperative pain is a disadvantage of using naloxone for the purpose of decreasing respiratory depression from preoperative narcotics. It can also cause tachycardia and hypertension, but is not associated with vomiting or addiction.

Questions

Q207

The nurse notes that the 80-year-old client who just arrived in the recovery room is shivering uncontrollably. The client experienced blood loss of 200 ml during a 4-hour surgery and has a preoperative history of mild acidosis. The nurse's priority interventions include:

1) removing wet linen from the bed, covering the client with a prewarmed blanket, monitoring temperature, and administering oxygen
2) allowing the shivering to take its natural course; shivering usually abates within the first few hours postoperatively
3) administering warm liquids to drink and allowing the client to breathe room air until the shivering eventually stops
4) notifying the physician and anesthesiologist immediately; this client is in grave danger of hypoxemia

*Your Own Answer*_____

Q208

The nurse's primary intervention for the postoperative client experiencing respiratory depression after being administered succinylcholine is:

1) administration of edrophonium to reverse the succinylcholine
2) administration of malathion to reverse the succinylcholine
3) administration of 100 percent oxygen at the rate of 6 L
4) continued mechanical ventilatory support

*Your Own Answer*_____

Correct Answers

A207

Answer 1 is the best choice. Shivering and hypothermia are not uncommon postoperatively, especially in the very young or very old client, during long surgical procedures, and with blood loss. Therefore, the nurse immediately initiates interventions for rewarming the client. Severe prolonged shivering can result in hypoxemia and even cardiac arrest. Therefore, answers 1 and 4 do not represent the best choices. Administering warm liquids and having the client breathe room air, as in answer 3, indicate that the nurse does not recognize the potential seriousness of postoperative shivering.

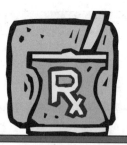

A208

Answer 4 is the best choice. Anticholinesterases, such as edrophonium, should never be given to reverse the neuromuscular blocking action of succinylcholine, as they prolong the effect of the drug. Malathion is a pesticide and is of no therapeutic benefit. Ventilatory support beyond oxygen administration should be given until normal respiratory function returns.

Questions

Q209

The nurse is aware that, in the average healthy person, a blood sample is obtained right after surgery in order to assess:

1) electrolytes and CBC
2) serum glucose level
3) arterial blood gases
4) all of the above

*Your Own Answer*_____

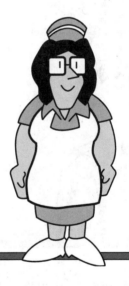

Q210

Immediately after surgery, the client always receives which of the following IV fluids:

1) RL, 500 ml/2 hrs
2) NS, 1000 ml/4 hrs
3) D5W, 500 ml/4 hrs
4) cannot be determined from given data

*Your Own Answer*_____

Correct Answers

A209

Answer 1 is the best choice. Answer 2 is not correct; serum glucose would only be assessed in the client with a prior diagnosis of diabetes. ABGs would be drawn only if an electrolyte imbalance were discovered after drawing a standard blood test (chem-20); therefore, answers 3 and 4 are also incorrect.

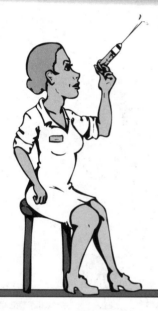

A210

Answer 4 is correct. There is no single standard postoperative IV therapy order. Factors that determine the type and amount of IV fluid to be infused include type of surgery, the client's preoperative status, and the client's response to the stress of surgery. Therefore, answers 1, 2, and 3 are not appropriate choices.

Questions

Q211

The recovery room nurse knows from experience that clients emerging from intraoperative anesthesia are at risk for delirium reaction. The nurse has noted that the type of client most likely to experience this reaction would be:

1) a calm, 30-year-old, normal-weight woman who underwent a scheduled Cesarean section for twins
2) a 25-year-old male with generalized anxiety disorder who underwent an emergency above-the-knee amputation
3) a depressed but otherwise physically healthy 65-year-old woman who underwent a cholecystectomy
4) a sometimes lethargic, 6-year-old, mentally retarded child who underwent a scheduled bilateral tonsillectomy

*Your Own Answer*_____

Q212

Common causes of hypertension during the postoperative period in an otherwise healthy client include which of the following:

1) the experience of pain
2) carbon dioxide retention
3) bladder distention
4) all of the above

*Your Own Answer*_____

Correct Answers

A211

Answer 2 is the best choice. Postoperative delirium most often occurs in highly nervous people who have experienced a sudden trauma. Therefore answers 1, 3, and 4 are not the best choices.

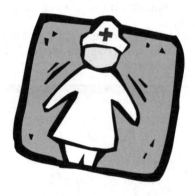

A212

Answer 4 is correct. All of these are common causes of transient hypertension postoperatively. Incisional pain can cause the client to avoid deep breathing and other methods that increase gas exchange—thereby increasing CO_2 retention—in the lungs. Bladder distension due to the inability to void may result in edema and increased blood pressure with the retention of water and especially sodium.

Questions

Q213

The nurse is creating a plan of care to ensure the physical and emotional comfort of a client returning from surgery. Which of the following nursing interventions is not intended to directly meet these goals:

1) covering the client with a prewarmed blanket and changing wet linens
2) administering adequate pain medication before the pain becomes severe
3) monitoring the client's oral and intravenous fluid intake and urine output
4) keeping the curtain drawn around the client's bed in the recovery room

*Your Own Answer*_____

Q214

The postoperative client in the recovery room needs to be reoriented to time and place:

1) at the beginning and end of the recovery room stay
2) only once as she/he emerges from the anesthesia
3) at frequent intervals while in the recovery room
4) only once at the time of transport to a regular unit

*Your Own Answer*_____

Correct Answers

A213

Answer 3 is the best choice. This is not a direct comfort measure. Answers 1, 2, and 4, therefore are not the best choices.

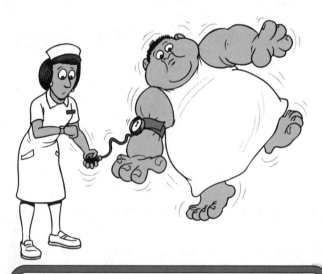

A214

Answer 3 is correct. Frequent reiteration of the time, date, and place by the recovery room nurse helps to decrease anxiety in the postanesthesia client. Therefore, answers 1, 2, and 4 are not the best choices.

Questions

Q215

The incidence of postoperative respiratory complications is lowest in clients having:

1) non-abdominothoracic surgery
2) thoracic surgery near the diaphragm
3) surgery inside the pelvic cavity
4) upper abdominal surgery

*Your Own Answer*_____

Q216

Postoperative atelectasis is usually:

1) self-limiting with an uneventful recovery
2) ongoing with a difficult, tenuous recovery
3) life-threatening, with frequent mortality
4) undiagnosed until other complications develop

*Your Own Answer*_____

Q217

Postoperative atelectasis results in shunting of the blood from the:

1) left to the right side of the heart
2) right to the left side of the heart
3) lower to the upper chambers of the heart
4) upper to the lower chambers of the heart

*Your Own Answer*_____

Correct Answers

A215

Answer 1 is the correct choice. Postoperative respiratory complications occur least often in surgery of the extremities, head, or neck. The greatest number of respiratory complications occur after surgery in the thoracic or abdominal cavity near the diaphragm muscle and somewhat less often after pelvic surgery.

A216

Answer 1 is correct. Although all postoperative clients experience some degree of atelectasis and therefore hypoxemia, atelectasis usually resolves by itself uneventfully. Therefore, answers 2, 3, and 4 are incorrect.

A217

Answer 2 is correct. Atelectasis causes pathological shunting of blood from the right side to the left side of the heart. Therefore, there is a decrease in the oxygenation blood that enters the systemic circulation, leading to hypoxemia. Answers 1, 3, and 4 are all incorrect.

Questions

Q218

Two days postsurgery, the nurse assesses a 65-year-old client who is complaining of chest pain, chills, and difficulty catching his breath. The nurse records a temperature of 102.6 degrees F and notes a productive cough and rust-colored sputum. On auscultation, rales are heard on inspiration and the client exhibits decreased breath sounds in the left lung. The nurse's priority action would be:

1) to perform tracheobronchial suctioning, chest percussion, and administer oxygen to reverse atelectasis
2) to draw blood specimens, obtain a urine sample, and monitor temperature to rule out septic shock
3) to obtain a sputum specimen and schedule a chest x-ray to rule out pneumonia
4) to assess the client's vital signs, intake and output, weight, and level of consciousness to rule out hypovolemic shock

*Your Own Answer*_____

Q219

The most frequent cause of hypovolemic shock in the postsurgical client is:

1) infection
2) psychosis
3) hemorrhage
4) hyperventilation

*Your Own Answer*_____

Correct Answers

A218

Answer 3 is the best choice. The elevated temperature and productive cough and rust-colored sputum should particularly alert the nurse to the possibility of postoperative pneumonia. These are not the presenting signs and symptoms of atelectasis, septic shock, or hypovolemic shock. Therefore, answers 1, 2, and 4 are not the best choices.

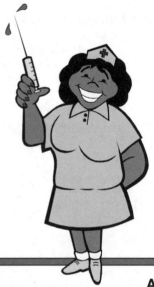

A219

Answer 3 is the correct choice. Dehydration also contributes to the risk for hypovolemic shock in the immediate postsurgical period.

Questions

Q220

In the client with postoperative hemorrhage, approximately 70 percent of the blood flow is shunted to the _____(a)_____ , while blood flow decreases in the _____(b)_____ .

(a)	(b)
1) kidneys	bowel, brain, skin, and liver
2) skin	bowel, liver, kidneys, and stomach
3) liver	kidneys, brain, skin, and stomach
4) brain	kidneys, bowel, skin, and liver

*Your Own Answer*_____

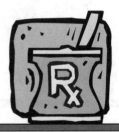

Q221

In the client experiencing a postoperative hemorrhage, cardiac output is maintained until what percent of the circulatory blood volume is lost:

1) 10 percent
2) 20 percent
3) 40 percent
4) 50 percent

*Your Own Answer*_____

Correct Answers

A220

Answer 4 is correct. Vasoconstriction shunts about 70 percent of the blood to the brain and away from the other organs. Therefore, answers 1, 2, and 3 are incorrect.

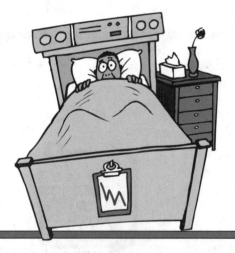

A221

Answer 2 is correct. With greater than 20 percent blood loss, the cells become deprived of oxygen, organs begin to dysfunction, and if the blood loss remains uncorrected organ failure, including heart, rapidly follows. Organs continue to function to some extent with 10 percent blood volume loss; therefore, answer 1 is not the best choice. Answers 3 and 4 represent situations in which organ function would not be supported.

Questions

Q222

Urinary output in the client with late-stage hypovolemic shock is:

1) 100ml/hour
2) 50-60ml/hour
3) 20-40 ml/hour
4) 10-30 ml/hour

*Your Own Answer*_____

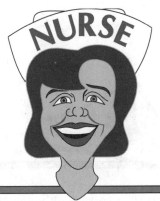

Q223

Most occurrences of septic shock are due to which type of microorganism:

1) fungi
2) viruses
3) gram-negative bacteria
4) gram-positive bacteria

*Your Own Answer*_____

Correct Answers

A222

Answer 3 is the best choice. Urinary output decreases greatly due to decreased blood flow to the kidneys as blood is shunted to the brain and vaso-constriction occurs elsewhere in the body. Normal urine output in an adult is between 1000-2000 ml/day (40-80 ml/hr). Therefore, an increase in urinary output to 200 ml/hr might indicate pathology, though other than hypovolemic shock; while an increase to 100 ml/hr is still within the range of normal. Therefore, answers 1, 2, and 4 are incorrect.

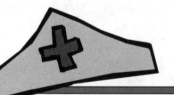

A223

Answer 3 is correct. Although other types of microorganisms may cause it, most cases of septic shock are due to gram-negative bacteria, such as *Escherichia coli, Klebsiella pneumoniae, Pseudomonas,* and others. Fungi, viruses, and gram-positive bacteria are less likely to be the cause of septic shock, often contracted in the OR. Answers 1, 2, and 4 are not good choices.

Questions

Q224

Priority interventions for the client experiencing hypovolemic shock do not include:

1) placing the client in the Trendelenburg position
2) placing the client flat in the bed
3) slightly elevating the client's legs
4) administering oxygen and covering the client with a blanket

*Your Own Answer*_____

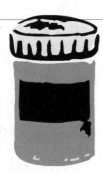

Q225

The majority of cases of gram-negative septicemia are caused by:

1) microorganisms brought in by visitors
2) microorganisms the client came in with
3) nosocomial infections
4) sterile procedures

*Your Own Answer*_____

Correct Answers

A224

Answer 1 is correct. The client should be placed flat in bed with legs slightly elevated to promote venous return and increase cardiac output. To conserve clients' energy, they are kept warm and given oxygen. The Trendelenburg position, with the head tilting downward is not recommended, as it may interfere with the client's efforts at respiration.

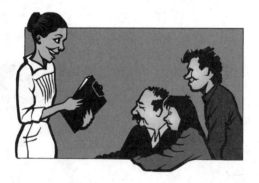

A225

Answer 3 is correct. Seventy percent of septic shock cases are due to hospital acquired infections. These are usually exceptionally virulent strains of gram-negative bacteria found on hospital linens, surfaces of furniture, and even within the air ducts of the hospital buildings. Answers 1, 2, and 4 are therefore incorrect.

Questions

Q226

The early stages of septic shock are recognized by which of the following clinical manifestations:
1) fever, chills, and flushed dry skin
2) moderately decreased urinary output and BP
3) increased pulse and respiration rates
4) all of the above

*Your Own Answer*_____

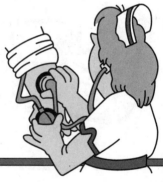

Q227

The most important preventive measure to lower the risk of septic shock is:
1) the use of aseptic technique, including frequent hand-washing
2) avoidance of contact between postoperative clients and their family
3) the least amount of contact between hospital staff and the client
4) the use of urinary catheters whenever possible to avoid stasis

*Your Own Answer*_____

Correct Answers

A226

Answer 4 is correct. These are all warning signs of the early "warm" stage of septic shock, which may last from 30 minutes to 12 hours before progressing to "cold shock" signs and symptoms.

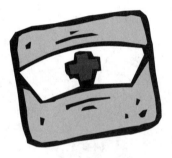

A227

Answer 1 is correct. Septic shock most often occurs due to nosocomial infections, obtained either during surgery or during postoperative sterile procedures not performed aseptically. It is unrealistic and/or dangerous for loved ones and hospital staff to avoid contact with the postoperative client. Urinary catheters should be used only when absolutely necessary due to their association with nosocomial infection. Therefore, answers 2, 3, and 4 are not the best choices.

Questions

Q228

Deep vein thrombosis occurs in the:

1) thoracic region and neck
2) upper extremities and neck
3) lower extremities and pelvis
4) abdominal region and chest

*Your Own Answer*_____

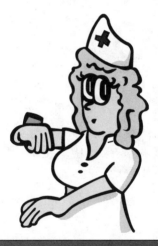

Q229

The nurse knows that the clients most at risk of developing a deep vein thrombosis (DVT) are those having undergone:

1) abdominal surgery
2) thoracic surgery
3) a fractured hip
4) a prostatectomy

*Your Own Answer*_____

Correct Answers

A228

Answer 3 is correct. Sluggish peripheral circulation most often causes stasis in the lower extremities and pelvic region, especially as a result of dehydration, shock, or congestive heart failure. Therefore, answers 1, 2, and 4 are not correct.

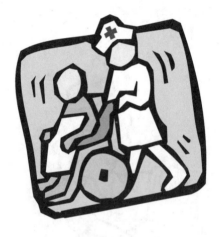

A229

Answer 3 is correct. Approximately 75 percent of those fracturing their hip will experience a DVT as a result. The lowest incidence is following abdominothoracic surgery. Following prostate surgery, about 50 percent will acquire a DVT.

Questions

Q230

The nurse is aware that in the client diagnosed with septicemia:

1) organism-specific antibiotic therapy will begin immediately
2) organism-specific antibiotic therapy will begin when C & S results are available
3) broad-spectrum antibiotic therapy will begin immediately
4) both answers 2 and 3

*Your Own Answer*_____

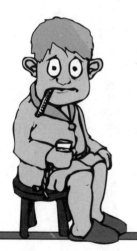

Q231

Which of the following is a contributing factor to the development of a deep vein thrombosis:

1) prolonged bed rest
2) obesity
3) cigarette smoking
4) each of the above

*Your Own Answer*_____

Correct Answers

A230

Answer 4 is correct. Intravenous fluids and broad-spectrum antibiotics should be given immediately upon diagnosis of septicemia, which constitutes a serious emergency. Once culture and sensitivity results are available, the order for antibiotic therapy will be specific for the type of microorganism causing the systemic infection. Answer 1 is therefore incorrect, and answers 2 and 3 by themselves do not constitute efficacious management of life-threatening septicemia.

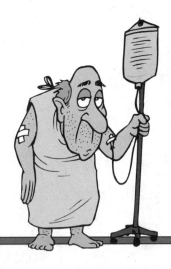

A231

Answer 4 is correct. Other risk factors include immobilization, advanced age, varicose veins, hip fracture, and certain major surgical procedures.

Questions

Q232

The major factors that influence the formation of a deep vein thrombosis (DVT) are least likely to include:

1) venous stasis
2) electrolyte imbalance
3) injury to the vein wall
4) hypercoagulability

*Your Own Answer*_____

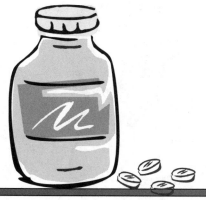

Q233

Deep vein thromboses usually develop:

1) 3 to 4 days after surgery and are always symptomatic
2) 7 to 10 days after surgery and are always symptomatic
3) 3 to 4 days after surgery and are always asymptomatic
4) 7 to 10 days after surgery and are often asymptomatic

*Your Own Answer*_____

Correct Answers

A232

Answer 2 is the correct choice. The other three factors, answers 1, 3, and 4, together are known as Virchow's Triad. One or more may cause a DVT.

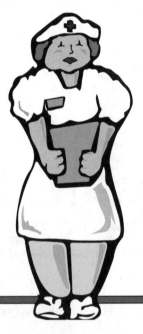

A233

Answer 4 is the correct choice. The majority of thrombi in the calf of the leg develop many days postsurgery and are asymptomatic, especially if the thrombus does not completely obstruct the flow of blood. Therefore, answers 1, 2, and 3 are not the best choices.

Questions

Q234

Hypercoagulability, one factor in the formation of a thrombus, is due to:

1) platelets
2) fibrin
3) antithrombin III
4) angiotensin II

*Your Own Answer*_____

Q235

If left untreated, a deep vein thrombosis (DVT) can lead to:

1) an embolus
2) a varicose vein
3) angina
4) an infection

*Your Own Answer*_____

Q236

The clinical sign which indicates a possible deep vein thrombosis is called:

1) a positive Babinski response
2) a negative Babinski response
3) a positive Homan's sign
4) a negative Homan's sign

*Your Own Answer*_____

Correct Answers

A234

Answer 3 is correct. Antithrombin III, a protein which circulates in the blood, inactivates thrombin and other clotting factors. Antithrombin III is part of the "coagulation cascade" that is set off by major surgery. A deficiency of platelets and fibrin leads to hypocoagulability. Therefore, answers 1 and 2 are incorrect. Angiotensin II is involved in the regulation of blood pressure, not blood clotting activity, making answer 4 also incorrect.

A235

Answer 1 is correct. Blood flowing past a formed thrombus may free it from the wall of the blood vessel. A detached thrombus is an embolus, which circulates until it is stopped somewhere in another blood vessel. A varicose vein, answer 2, is simply an enlarged, usually twisted superficial vein and is generally not life-threatening. Angina refers to chest pain due to insufficient oxygen to the heart, and is not usually directly related to a DVT; therefore answer 3 is incorrect. Answer 4, is not a good choice as DVTs do not lead directly to infection.

A236

Answer 3 is the correct choice. A positive Homan's sign, that is, calf pain on dorsiflexion of the foot, is a reasonable indicator that follow up with Doppler ultrasound is warranted to rule out a DVT. Babinski's response is an indication of upper motor neuron disease. Therefore, answers 1, 2, and 4 are incorrect.

Questions

Q237

Immediately upon diagnosis of a deep vein thrombosis (DVT) in a bedridden client, the nurse knows that the plan of care will include which of the following nursing actions:

1) frequent, vigorous ambulation of the client
2) active range-of-motion exercise of the affected leg
3) an antiembolic stocking for the affected leg only
4) measurement of each leg circumference q day

*Your Own Answer*_____

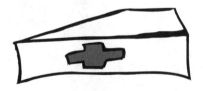

Q238

In a client with a deep vein thrombosis, the nurse is aware that the affected leg is wrapped with an elastic support bandage:

1) from the toes up, after elevating the feet
2) from the calf down, after elevating the feet
3) above the knee, after dangling the feet
4) and not unwrapped until the end of treatment

*Your Own Answer*_____

Correct Answers

A237

Answer 4 is the best choice. Both legs are measured each day in order to detect swelling, which could compromise the circulation distal to the DVT. In addition, the nurse should assess the motor and neurological function of the feet q shift. In a bedridden client, immediate ambulation is unrealistic. Active ROM could cause the DVT to be dislodged, creating an embolus. Antiembolic stockings should be applied to the unaffected leg only at first, and then once the client is walking, applied to the affected leg as well.

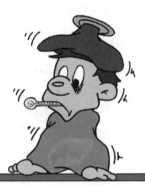

A238

Answer 1 is the best choice. Wrapping the affected leg in this manner encourages venous return most efficiently. The affected leg is not wrapped above the knee to avoid putting pressure on the popliteal vein. Wrapping the leg from the calf downward encourages the engorgement of leg veins. The client is instructed to wear the bandage at all times, but it should be removed and rewrapped once per shift.

Questions

Which of the following medications is least likely to be ordered for the client upon diagnosis with deep vein thrombosis (DVT):

I.   warfarin
II. heparin
Ill. vitamin K
IV. colace

1) I, II, and III
2) II, III, and IV
3) I, II, and IV
4) all of the above

*Your Own Answer*_____

The nurse is performing preoperative teaching with Ms. Cunningham, who is scheduled for pelvic surgery the next day. The teaching includes effective methods for the prevention of a deep vein thrombosis. The nurse knows that Ms. Cunningham has misunderstood the instructions when she states:

1) "I will get out of bed with assistance and begin to walk as soon after surgery as possible."
2) "I will perform deep-breathing exercises every 2 hours as soon after surgery as possible."
3) "I will perform range-of-motion exercises every 2 hours in order to keep mobility in my joints."
4) "I will massage my lower legs vigorously every 2 hours in order to avoid leg cramps."

*Your Own Answer*_____

Correct Answers

A239

The correct answer is 3. Heparin and warfarin are given immediately upon diagnosis of a DVT, though the warfarin has a delayed action of 5 to 7 days. Warfarin is often continued after the thrombus is dissolved, if the client is at risk for development of another thrombus. Colace is also given to soften stools and therefore to help the client avoid straining. Pressure due to straining can dislodge a thrombus, sending it out into the circulation as a more dangerous embolus. Vitamin K is an antihemorrhagic factor that aids blood clotting, and would therefore not be used therapeutically here.

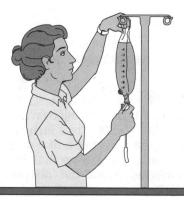

A240

Answer 4 is the correct choice. Massaging the calves of the legs may break a thrombus up into fragments, thereby releasing it into the circulation as an embolus. The other three methods, answers 1, 2, and 3, are appropriate interventions in the prevention of a DVT.

Questions

The nurse is aware that the reason for the administration of heparin in a client with a pulmonary embolus is to:

1) dissolve the existing clot
2) prevent embolus recurrence
3) potentiate the warfarin
4) alleviate severe chest pain

*Your Own Answer*_____

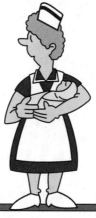

Q242

The nurse is aware that the best preventive nursing interventions to lower the risk of developing a pulmonary embolus are the same as those to prevent:

1) deep vein thrombosis
2) myocardial infarction
3) septic shock
4) viral pneumonia

*Your Own Answer*_____

Correct Answers

A241

The correct choice is answer 2. Heparin has no fibrinolytic ability, and so cannot dissolve the existing clot. Therefore, answer 1 is incorrect. If managed carefully, most clots dissolve on their own. Heparin does not potentiate warfarin; however, warfarin is also useful in the prevention of future thrombi. Answer 3 is therefore not the best choice. Nitroglycerine, not heparin, might be given to alleviate severe chest pain related to a potential MI; therefore, answer 4 is incorrect.

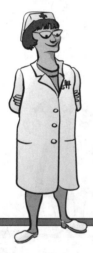

A242

Answer 1 is correct. Since the lower extremity or pelvic veins are the most common starting point for a pulmonary embolus, the preventive measures are the same as those for deep vein thrombosis. These include, among others, deep breathing exercises and elevation of the legs to encourage venous return, the use of antiembolic support stockings, and early ambulation. Answers 2, 3, and 4 are therefore not good choices.

Questions

Q243

Positioning of the client who survives a pulmonary embolus includes:

1) the legs elevated 10-15 degrees and the rest of the body supine
2) the legs elevated 10-15 degrees and the head of the bed 30-45 degrees
3) placing the client in the Trendelenburg position
4) placing the client's entire body in the supine position

*Your Own Answer*_____

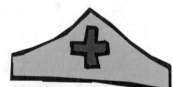

Q244

The nurse knows that it is dangerous to administer streptokinase to the client with a massive, life-threatening pulmonary embolus if the client:

1) has a history of cardiovascular disease
2) is allergic to penicillin-type medications
3) had surgery or a biopsy in the past 12 days
4) has a history of hepatic or renal insufficiency

*Your Own Answer*_____

Correct Answers

A243

Answer 2 is the best choice. The client placed in the supine or Trendelenberg positions will have difficulty attaining full expansion of the chest. With the head of the bed in semi-Fowler's position, breathing will be facilitated by good chest expansion. Slightly elevating the foot of the bed encourages venous return.

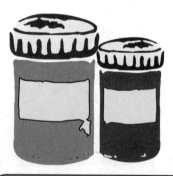

A244

Answer 3 is correct. The thrombolytic agent streptokinase could cause bleeding at the site of the biopsy or surgical incision. The situations in answers 1, 2, or 4 do not present contraindications to the use of this drug.

Questions

Q245

Hiccoughs are caused by uncontrollable contractions of the diaphragm, which is innervated by the:

1) vagus nerve
2) pectoral nerves
3) axillary nerve
4) phrenic nerves

*Your Own Answer*_____

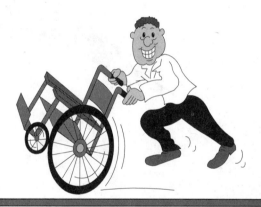

Q246

Mrs. Brown is a 78-year-old female, with an 18-year history of rheumatoid arthritis. Which of the following is least likely to be noted during Mrs. Brown's physical examination in the early stages of diagnosis:

1) inflammation
2) swelling
3) can only occur in children
4) possibly warmth and reduced motion

*Your Own Answer*_____

Correct Answers

A245

Answer 4 is correct. The phrenic nerves derive from the cervical plexus and innervate the diaphragm. The vagus nerve, or 10th cranial nerve, innervates the stomach, liver, lungs, kidney, and spleen, among other organs. The pectoral nerve does not exist. The axillary nerve innervates parts of the upper arm and shoulder. Therefore, answers 1, 2, and 3 are incorrect.

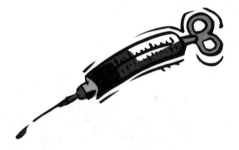

A246

The correct answer is 3. Rheumatoid arthritis can occur at any age. Answers 1, 2, and 4 occur because the joints have a soft, spongy feeling due to the synovial thickening and inflammation.

Questions

Q247

Which of the following treatment goals for Mrs. Brown's rheumatoid arthritis would least likely occur:

1) short-term adherence to prescribed treatment modalities
2) reduce pain
3) minimize stiffness and swelling
4) maintain mobility

*Your Own Answer*_____

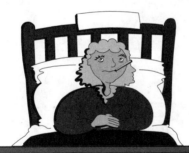

Q248

Mrs. Brown sustained a stress fracture of the right tibia and a hard cast is applied. While monitoring for complications, the nurse should assess the extremity for:

1) warmth
2) numbness
3) skin desquamation
4) generalized discomfort

*Your Own Answer*_____

Correct Answers

A247

The correct answer is 1. Rheumatoid arthritis is a chronic disease and requires continuous long term adherence to prescribed treatment modalities. Answers 2, 3, and 4 are all treatment goals designed to maintain optimal mobility.

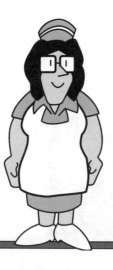

A248

The correct answer is 2. Numbness is a neurologic sign that should be reported immediately, because it indicates pressure on the nerves and blood vessels. Answer 1, warmth, is a normal reaction to a new cast. Answer 3, results from inadequate skin care, and answer 4 is incorrect because some degree of discomfort is expected following cast application.

Questions

Q249

Mrs. Brown is placed on a slow-acting medication called Plaquenil Sulfate. Which of the following statements would least likely be included in the nurse's instructions:

1) to use sunglasses in bright sunlight to decrease photophobia
2) that urine may turn rust to brown
3) take medication any time during the day
4) oral medication to be stored in tight, light-resistant container at room temperature

*Your Own Answer*_____

Q250

While preparing Mrs. Brown's medication, the nurse notes that the physican has halved the usual dosage of the drug. She should:

1) administer the drug
2) contact the doctor and verify dosage ordered
3) chart that on overdosage was ordered
4) check the orders with several other staff nurses before administering the drug

*Your Own Answer*_____

Correct Answers

A249

The correct answer is 3. Medication is to be administered at the same time each day to maintain drug level. Answers 1, 2, and 4 are correct instruction for patient/family teaching.

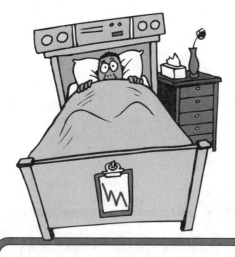

A250

Answer 2 is correct. Whenever the nurse is going to administer a medication and a problem noted, the nurse should contact the doctor for verification and/or clarification. Answers 1, 3, and 4 are all incorrect because only the physician or covering doctor can order medication changes.

Questions

Mrs. Kelly has anemia due to chemotherapy and the doctor has started her on epogen 10,000 units every Monday, Wednesday, and Friday. The visiting nurse would administer the medication:

1) intramuscularly
2) in rectal suppository form
3) subcutaneously
4) sublingually

*Your Own Answer*_____

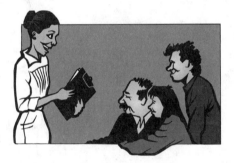

Q252

Mr. Reilly is an insulin-dependent diabetic, who suddenly shows symptoms of a hypoglycemic reaction. Which of the following groups of symptoms would be indicative of this reaction:

1) rapid deep respiration, acetone on breath, drowsiness
2) chest pains, nausea, sweats
3) nausea, vomiting, visual disturbances
4) restlessness, profuse sweating, trembling

*Your Own Answer*_____

Correct Answers

A251

Answer 3 is correct. This medication is administered either subcutaneously or intravenously. Answers 1, 2, and 4 are incorrect routes of administration.

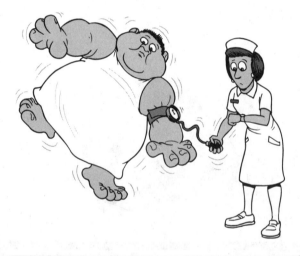

A252

Answer 4 is correct. The symptoms of hypoglycemia included in answer 4 are the result of a drop in blood sugar. Profuse perspiration is caused by the release of epinephrine due to the decrease in blood sugar. Answer 1 includes symptoms of hyperglycemia; answer 2 may be indicating possible myocardial infarction, and answer 3 may be indicative of a number of disease processes.

Questions

Q253

Mr. Murphy has a history of hypertension. The doctor has placed him on a sodium-restricted diet. Which groups of foods may he consume:

1) smoked salmon, fresh fruit, canned vegetables, apple juice
2) sweet butter, chicken, puffed rice, ginger ale
3) tomato juice, cheddar cheese, fresh fruit, and fresh vegetables
4) chicken, saltine crackers, ice cream

*Your Own Answer*_____

Q254

Prednisone, a corticosteroid, is ordered for a patient with an exacerbation of Chronic Obstructive Pulmonary Disease. When administering the first dose, the nurse should stress that this drug:

1) will prevent the patient from getting an infection
2) is not a curative but does cause a suppression in the inflammatory process
3) may be stopped at any time
4) may decrease the patient's appetite causing weight loss

*Your Own Answer*_____

Correct Answers

A253

Answer 2 is correct. A person on a sodium restricted diet should avoid canned fruits and vegetables since they contain sodium; smoked foods, cheeses, and tomato juice also contain high percentages of sodium.

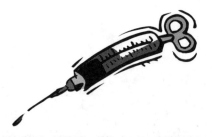

A254

The correct answer is 2. Prednisone decreases inflammation by suppressing the migration of polymorphanuclear leukocytes and fibroblasts. It also increases capillary permeability. This is a symptomatic treatment, not a curative one. 1) the drug suppresses the immune response and increases the potential for infection; 3) drug may not be stopped abruptly or adrenal crisis can result ; 4) the appetite is increased and weight gain may result from this or fluid retention.

Questions

Q255

When obtaining a health history on a newly-diagnosed, non-insulin dependent diabetic, the nurse should expect the patient to present the classic signs and symptoms of diabetes mellitus, such as:

1) polyuria, irritability, polydipsia
2) polydipsia, nocturia, weight loss
3) polydipsia, polyuria, polyphagia
4) polyphagia, polyuria, confusion

*Your Own Answer*_____

Q256

A patient is diagnosed as an insulin-dependent diabetic. The doctor orders 8 units of regular insulin subcutaneously every morning before breakfast. Which of the following outcomes would the nurse least likely expect:

1) onset 1/2 - 1 hour with 2-4 hour peak and 6-8 hour duration
2) onset 1-2 hours with 6-8 hours peak and 12-14 hour duration
3) clear appearance
4) compatible mix with all insulin preparations

*Your Own Answer*_____

Correct Answers

A255

The correct answer is 3. Excessive thirst, frequent urination, and excessive hunger are caused by the body's inability to correctly metabolize glucose.

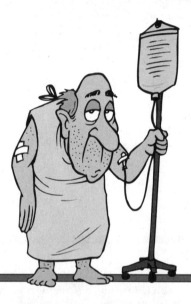

A256

Answer 2 is correct. Insulin preparations of intermediate action have onset 1-2 hours, peak 6-8, and duration between 12-16 hours depending on preparation. 1) onset 1/2 - 1 hour, peak 24 hours with duration 6-8 hours or 8-10 hours depending on preparation. 3) insulin (regular), regular Iletin and regular Iletin U-500 all have a clear appearance. 4) insulin regular is compatible with all insulin preparations.

Questions

Q257

Proper foot care is important to all diabetics. The nurse should give instruction to patients with non-insulin dependent diabetes to:

1) wash feet daily with mild soap and water and dry thoroughly
2) to cut corns and calluses
3) always wear shoes and use natural fiber socks
4) wear slightly larger shoes and nylon socks

*Your Own Answer*_____

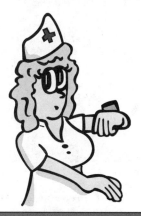

Q258

A public health nurse is implementing a screening program for scoliosis. The most appropriate site would be in a:

1) preschool day care center
2) middle school
3) senior high school
4) well-baby clinic

*Your Own Answer*_____

Correct Answers

A257

Answer 3 is correct. Wearing shoes protects the feet; shoes should fit well and be worn with cotton or wool socks to cushion the feet and absorb perspiration; 1) feet should be washed daily with mild soap and water and dried thoroughly between toes using pressure. Rubbing vigorously is apt to break the delicate skin; 2) under no circumstances should skin become irritated. Cutting or tearing calluses and corns causes irritation and risk of infection; 4) shoes that don't fit well will create friction and cause blisters, sores and calluses. Nylon isn't a natural fiber and promotes perspiration.

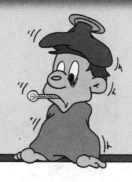

A258

Answer 2 is correct. Preadolescents and young adolescents are most at risk and can be most successfully treated. 1) 80 percent of patients with idiopathic scoliosis are not preschoolers, they are preadolescents and young adolescents; 3) some students with scoliosis might be identified, but it may be too late for adequate treatment; 4) scoliosis would not be identifiable in children at this age.

 Take Test-Readiness Quiz 3 on CD
(to review questions 171–258)

Questions

A public health nurse is visiting a patient with chronic obstructive pulmonary disease who is primarily bed bound. The nurse notes upon assessment a small decubitus ulcer on the sacral area. The nurse should plan to deal with this problem by:

1) keeping the area dry
2) applying moist dressing
3) providing a low-calorie diet
4) keeping the patient on the right side

*Your Own Answer*_____

A public health nurse is lecturing at a local high school on sex education, specifically Herpes genitalis. The nurse should tell the students that:

1) the disease is not transmitted via fomites such as toilet seats
2) Herpes genitalis is curable with penicillin
3) the disease is generally painless in women
4) herpes genitalis causes both local and systemic reactions

*Your Own Answer*_____

Correct Answers

A259

Answer 1 is correct. This promotes tissue regeneration and prevents creating a moist area conducive to infection. 2) A moist dressing creates a warm, moist protein-containing medium that is ideal for growing pathogens; 3) a high caloric diet is appropriate to provide energy for tissue repair; 4) placing the patient in one position will promote development of additional decubitus ulcers.

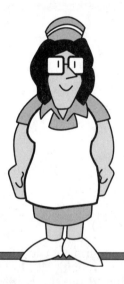

A260

Answer 4 is correct. Fever, headache and malaise may accompany local reactions. 1) Although uncommon, a virus can survive for short periods of time on toilet seats or locker benches; 2) Herpes is of viral origin; there is no cure and antibiotics are ineffective; 3) vesicles on genitalia rupture, causing painful ulcerations.

Questions

Mr. Reilly is extremely upset after a stressful event and is rambling with rapid speech. A therapeutic technique that the nurse can use is:

1) silence
2) focusing
3) touch
4) summarizing

*Your Own Answer*_____

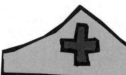

Q262

A nurse working at a local crisis and intervention center attempts to remain objective and supportive of patients in crisis. The nurse uses imagination and determination to project herself into the patients' emotions. The nurse would best accomplish this by using the technique known as:

1) empathy
2) sympathy
3) projection
4) acceptance

*Your Own Answer*_____

Correct Answers

A261

Answer 2 is correct. The nurse attempts to concentrate or focus the client's communication on one specific episode. 1) Silence would prolong the rambling speech; 3) touch would invade the patient's space and would do nothing to help focus the client's communications; 4) summarizing would be impossible until the concern is identified and explored.

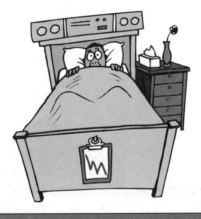

A262

Answer 1 is correct. Empathy is the ability to project one's self into another's emotions and to share the emotion and state of mind. 2) Sympathy is a shared expression of sorrow over an imagined loss or real loss; 3) projection is an unconscious defense and not a therapeutic technique; 4) acceptance is just that. The nurse would accept the patients' emotions and not project herself into the patients' emotions.

Questions

Q263

Three days after the stressful event, Mr. Reilly can no longer remember what he was worried about. The inability to recall the situation is an example of the defense mechanism of:

1) denial
2) repression
3) regression
4) dissociation

*Your Own Answer*_____

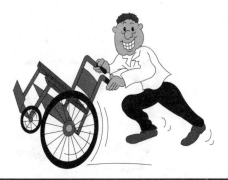

Q264

A patient brought into the emergency room is suspected of and demonstrating the symptoms associated with opiate overdose. The nurse would expect the doctor to prescribe:

1) naloxone (Narcan)
2) methadone (Dolophine HCL)
3) epinephrine (adrenalin chloride)
4) amphetamine

*Your Own Answer*_____

Correct Answers

A263

Answer 2 is correct. The patient's inability to re-call is an example of repression. It is an uncon-scious and involuntary forgetting of painful events and conflicts. 1) There is nothing to dem-onstrate that denial, an unconscious refusal to admit that an unacceptable behavior or idea, has occurred; 3) there is nothing to demonstrate that regression, to return to an earlier, more comfort-able developmental level, has occurred; 4) there is nothing to demonstrate that dissociation, the separation and detachment of emotional affect and significance from a particular idea, situation, or incident, has occurred.

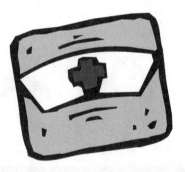

A264

Answer 1 is correct. The drug is a narcotic antago-nist that displaces narcotics from receptors in the brain, reversing respiratory depression. 2) This is a synthetic opiate that causes CNS depression; 3) this drug would have no effect on respiratory depression related to the presence of an overdose of a narcotic; 4) same as answer 3.

Questions

Mary Smith is a 62-year-old female, who w
mitted to the hospital emergency room pr
ing with the signs and symptoms of a potassium
deficit. She is started on a potassium solution
drip. In order to prevent cardiac arrest, the rate
of drip per hour is usually no more than:

1) 45 meq
2) 20 meq
3) 30 meq
4) 40 meq

*Your Own Answer*_____

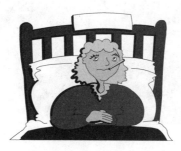

Q266

Mary Smith's potassium deficit is thought to be
related to poor dietary habits. She is instructed
to eat foods high in potassium. Which food has
the highest content?

1) banana (one medium)
2) cantaloupe (1/2 5" diameter)
3) wheat germ (100 gm)
4) prunes (raw, five large)

*Your Own Answer*_____

A265

Answer 2 is correct. If potassium is infused too rapidly, cardiac arrest may result due to the effect of potassium on the cardiac muscle. 1) Too rapid an infusion of potassium can lead to cardiac arrest due to the effect of potassium on cardiac muscle and severe pain can develop along the vein used for the potassium infusion; 3) and 4) same as answer one.

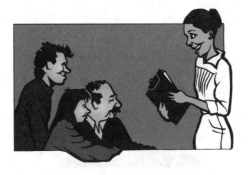

A266

Answer 3 is correct. Wheat germ = 737 mg; answers 1), 2) and 4) are all good sources of potassium but wheat germ is higher. Banana = 628 mg, cantaloupe = 230 mg, and prunes = 300 mg.

Questions

Q267

Mrs. Brown is a 32-year-old female admitted to the hospital for an appendectomy. She is to receive spinal anesthesia. Which of the following is the least possible complication or discomfort the nurse can expect?

1) nausea and vomiting
2) headache
3) hypotension
4) hypertension

*Your Own Answer*_____

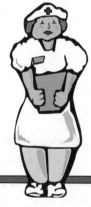

Q268

Mrs. Green, a 54-year-old female, was recently diagnosed as an insulin-dependent diabetic. Which is not one of the four cardinal symptoms of diabetes:

1) polyuria
2) polydipsia
3) weight gain
4) polyphagia

*Your Own Answer*_____

Correct Answers

A267

Answer 4 is correct. Paralysis of vasomotor nerves usually occurs shortly after induction of anesthesia and hypotension may occur, not hypertension. 1) Occurs mainly during abdominal surgery due to traction placed on various structures within the abdomen or at times due to hypotension; 2) cerebral spinal fluid is lost through dural hole; leakage of fluid and loss of cushioning effect increased by use of a large spinal needle and or poor hydration; 3) see answer 4.

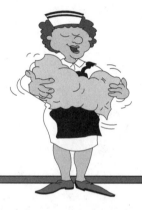

A268

Answer 3 is correct. Weight loss occurs—not weight gain—because glucose is not available to the cells; fat and protein stores are broken down and used for energy. 1) Polyuria occurs since water is not reabsorbed by the renal tubules because of the osmotic activity of glucose; 2) polyuria causes severe dehydration which in turn causes polydipsia (extreme thirst); 4) polyphagia causes tissue breakdown and wasting which creates a state of starvation which compels the stricken individual to eat voraciously.

Questions

Q269

Mr. Jackson is placed on a 2-gm sodium diet due to hypertension. Which of the following would indicate that Mr. Jackson understands his diet when he chooses:

1) sardines on crackers with salted tops and diet soda
2) turkey, tomato and lettuce on white bread with black coffee
3) frankfurter and sauerkraut on roll and beer
4) bacon, lettuce, and tomato on white bread with diet soda

*Your Own Answer*_____

Q270

A patient is admitted to the hospital with a diagnosis of congestive heart failure. The doctor orders daily weights. Which of the following is least advisable in obtaining an accurate reading of the patient's weight:

1) make sure patient isn't touching anything while standing on scale
2) that scale is on a hard flat level surface
3) weigh patient undressed or in light weight gown at same time each day
4) weigh patient immediately after a meal

*Your Own Answer*_____

Correct Answers

A269

Answer 2 is correct. Turkey, tomato, and lettuce on white bread and diet soda are all low in sodium content; 1), 3), and 4) are all high in sodium. Smoked and processed foods such as sardines, frankfurters, and bacon are all high in sodium. Salt shouldn't be used in food preparation at stove or on table.

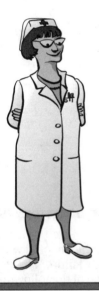

A270

Answer 4 is correct. Patient weights increase directly after meals due to food and fluid intake, size and portion; 1), 2), and 3) are all advisable in order to obtain an accurate reading.

Questions

Q271

A nurse working in a hospital would expect which of the following medications to be locked in a cabinet in the medication room? Any preparation containing:

1) cortisone
2) codeine
3) caffeine
4) quinine

*Your Own Answer*_____

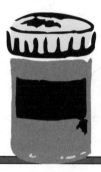

Q272

Following a pharmacy delivery on the hospital floor, the nurse separating the medical supplies would refrigerate which of the following:

1) petroleum jelly
2) piperazine adipate
3) glycerin suppositories
4) aspirin tablets

*Your Own Answer*_____

Correct Answers

A271

Answer 2 is correct. Codeine is a controlled substance with a functional class of narcotic analgesics that is addictive and requires close monitoring and stored under lock and key. 1) Cortisone is not a controlled substance; its functional class is corticosteroid synthetic. 3) Caffeine is not a controlled substance; its functional class is an analeptic. 4) Quinine is not a controlled substance; its functional class is antimalarial.

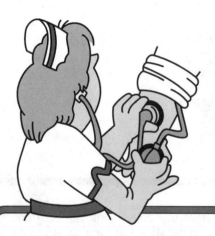

A272

Answer 3 is correct. Glycerin suppositories need to be stored in a cool environment but not frozen; 1) petroleum jelly storage is at room temperature; 2) piperazine adipate should be stored in a tight container at room temperature; 4) aspirin is stored at room temperature.

Questions

Q273

A home health nurse notes upon receiving a patient's medications that some of the prescription bottles have clear tape over the labels. The nurse would instruct the patient that to cover a typed label on a medicine bottle with clear tape is:

1) inadvisable, the tape may have a chemical reaction on the drug
2) advisable, the label will become waterproof and the printing on it will remain legible
3) inadvisable, the tape will make the printing on the label unchangeable
4) advisable, the tape will prevent the bottle from breaking

*Your Own Answer*_____

Q274

A nurse at a public awareness seminar would make people aware that a service that the American Heart Association does not offer is:

1) support of research in cardiovascular disease
2) programs for public and professional education on cardiovascular disease
3) information about and referral to community resources
4) clinics for the treatment of patients with cardiovascular disease

*Your Own Answer*_____

Correct Answers

A273

Answer 2 is correct. Many patients on home care store their medication in the kitchen and bathroom by sinks. Wet labels, whether from handling with wet hands or dropping on wet surfaces, become difficult to read and increase the risk of medication error; 1) tape adhesive will not permeate plastic and contaminate the medication; 3) medication labels should never be tampered with, that increases the risk of error when medicating; 4) any broken container containing medication should be replaced and medication properly disposed of.

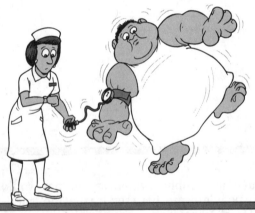

A274

Answer 4 is correct. Clinics for the treatment of a patient with cardiovascular disease would be by the referral of his/her physician after complete examination and testing; 1),2), and 3) are all services provided by the American Heart Association.

Questions

Mrs. Jones was discharged home from the hospital following an acute myocardial infarction. The physician has ordered a visiting home care nurse to visit two times a week for two weeks. When planning to visit the patient in her home for the first time, the nurse should be aware that the primary purpose of this visit is to:

1) gain information and build rapport
2) analyze the health needs of the family
3) teach the patient about her illness
4) give information regarding available health facilities in the community

*Your Own Answer*_____

Ms. Logan is a 24-year-old female taking oral contraceptives for the first time. The nurse provides written literature in addition to verbal instructions. The nurse instructs the patient to stop taking the contraceptive and report to the physician immediately if she experiences:

1) vertigo and nausea
2) weight loss
3) hypotension and amenorrhea
4) headaches and visual disturbances

*Your Own Answer*_____

Correct Answers

A275

Answer 1 is correct. Gaining information and building a rapport are the primary purpose of the first visit in order to assess patient needs, ability, and willingness to participate in self-care and promote comfort level and trust; 2) first priority is the patient; family health needs are not addressed, family members who act as caregivers are assessed for willingness and capability. 3) Disease processes and limitations are addressed as rapport and trust develop and limitations are established. 4) Patient is given information regarding health facilities in the community as discharge nears and by advice of physician and nurse reinforcement.

A276

Answer 4 is correct. Headaches may indicate hypertension or a cardiovascular event. Visual disturbances may indicate neuroocular lesions that are associated with the use of oral contraceptives; 1) vertigo and nausea are side effects and dosage may have to be adjusted if persistent or uncomfortable for patient; 2) weight gain, not loss, occurs because of edema; 3) hypotension and amenorrhea do not occur; hypertension may occur with oral contraceptives and subside when they are discontinued.

Questions

Q277

Proper nursing instructions to a patient who is breastfeeding her baby and has developed nipples that are sore and cracked is:

1) apply continuous ice packs to her nipples
2) take her analgesic medication as ordered
3) discontinue breast feeding for a few days
4) expose her nipples to the air several times a day

*Your Own Answer*_____

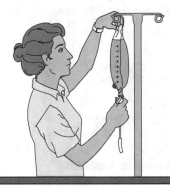

Q278

Mr. Brown, a 56-year-old male, was admitted to the medical floor with a diagnosis of right-sided cardiovascular accident and is right-handed. The task that will probably present the most difficulty would be:

1) eating meals
2) dressing every morning
3) writing letters
4) combing his hair

*Your Own Answer*_____

Correct Answers

A277

Answer 4 is correct. Exposing the nipples to the air several times a day hardens the nipples and reduces soreness; 1) continuous ice packs would cause vasoconstriction and cause milk suppression; 2) an ordered analgesic would reduce the soreness but not dry and harden the nipples; 3) discontinuation of breast feeding for a few days would inhibit lactation since the breasts must be emptied regularly for milk production to continue.

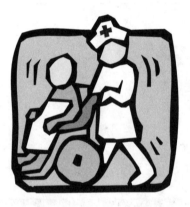

A278

Answer 2 is correct. Many aspects of dressing require movement of both sides of the body and both hands especially with closures on clothing; 1) the patient can continue to use the right hand to perform this activity; 3) and 4) same as answer 1.

Questions

Mr. Ball was admitted to the hospital emergency room presenting with a temperature of 101.6 degrees F orally, productive cough, and chills for the past three days. The nurse percusses an area of dullness over the right posterior lower lobe. Considering the signs and symptoms presented and her assessment, the nurse is aware the findings may be indicative of

1) pleurisy
2) bronchitis
3) pneumonia
4) emphysema

*Your Own Answer*_____

A child is admitted to the pediatric emergency room with multiple bruises and abrasions with vague answers to questions on occurrence. The nurse suspects the child has been abused; the nurse's primary responsibility must be to:

1) treat the child's injuries
2) confirm the suspected child abuse
3) protect the child from any further abuse
4) have the child examined by the physician

*Your Own Answer*_____

Correct Answers

A279

Answer 3 is correct. The findings indicate an infectious process in the lung; 1) a pleurisy patient's signs and symptoms would present with pain in the lower lobe at the height of inspiration and a pleural friction rub; 2) fever and chills may occur later in bronchitis, the signs and symptoms are irritating cough, chest pains, and shortness of breath; 4) emphysema signs and symptoms would be barrel chest, resonance on percussions, and thick tenacious sputum.

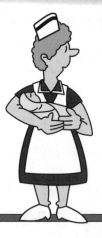

A280

Answer 3 is correct. Most injuries to abused children aren't life threatening; protection takes priority over immediate treatment; 1) the physician's primary responsibility is treatment of medical injuries; 2) an accurate diagnosis of child abuse takes time and must be fully investigated; 4) the nurse is often the first individual to see the abused child and must establish protection even before the physician arrives.

Questions

Q281

Ms. Murphy was admitted to the hospital with a diagnosis of hemolytic anemia. Which of the following would the nurse be least likely to expect:

1) jaundice
2) splenomegaly, hepatomegaly and hyperplasia of bone marrow
3) autonomic dysreflexia
4) cholelithiasis

*Your Own Answer*_____

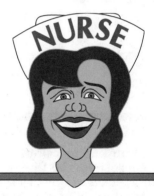

Q282

Which of the following is the least possible sign and symptom of the disease process polycythemia vera a nurse would expect to see in the patient:

1) enlarged liver or spleen
2) congestive heart failure
3) ruddy complexion and dusky redness of mucosa
4) severe pruritus

*Your Own Answer*_____

Correct Answers

A281

Answer 3 is correct. Autonomic dysreflexia is not related to hemolytic anemia. It is a potentially life threatening complication that occurs to spinal cord injured patients during a bladder training program or if their urinary drainage system becomes obstructed; 1) jaundice occurs due to abnormally large amounts of bilirubin that accumulate within the blood, owing to excessive destruction of erythrocytes; 2) all of these occur due to reticuloendothelial elements within the spleen, liver, and bone marrow. It becomes hyperactive because of the increased demand upon them to phagocytize defective erythrocytes. 4) Cholelithiasis occurs due to excessive accumulation of bilirubin due to destruction of erythrocytes and leads to development of pigment stones within the gallbladder.

A282

Answer 4 is correct. Severe pruritus is an early sign and symptom of Hodgkin's Disease with the cause unknown; 1) enlarged liver or spleen occurs due to large numbers of erythrocytes that collect within the liver and spleen; increased volume of blood within the portal circulation also causes organ congestion; 2) congestive heart failure occurs due to increased blood volume and viscosity that increases the work of the heart leading to failure; 3) ruddy complexion and dusky redness of mucosa occur due to the great volume of blood and causes congestion of capillaries supplying skin and mucous membranes.

Questions

Q283

Mr. Day receives an intravenous push of Lasix 40 mg during an episode of congestive heart failure. You observe his output by Foley catheter expecting to see a diuresis:

1) within five minutes
2) within 1/2 to one hour
3) within two to four hours
4) within four to six hours

*Your Own Answer*_____

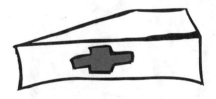

Q284

A nurse working on an oncology floor would recognize that which one of the following is not an example of a malignant epithelium neoplasm:

1) carcinoma
2) adenocarcinoma
3) squamous cell carcinoma
4) papilloma

*Your Own Answer*_____

Correct Answers

A283

Answer 1 is correct. Lasix push of intravenous onset of action is within 5 minutes; acts on loop of Henle by increasing excretions of chloride, sodium; 2), 3) and 4) are all incorrect. Lasix onset of action intravenously is within 5 minutes, peak action 30 minutes, duration of action 2 hours.

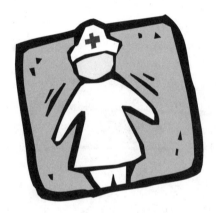

A284

Answer 4 is correct. Papilloma is a benign neoplasm of epithelium tissue origin; 1), 2), and 3) are all examples of malignant epithelium neoplasms. Carcinoma and squamous cell carcinoma are from skin and mucous membrane tissue origin and adenocarcinoma is from gland tissue origin.

Questions

Q285

Mrs. Marris has a history of arthritis and takes aspirin 325 mg 1-2 tablets every 4-6 hours as needed for pain. When assessing the patient it is important to know that an overdose of aspirin may cause:

1) dry skin
2) tinnitus
3) restlessness
4) tachypnea

*Your Own Answer*_____

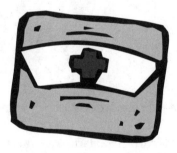

Q286

A nurse working in a hospital emergency room would be aware the disease not caused by a virus is:

1) malaria
2) poliomyelitis
3) rabies
4) yellow fever

*Your Own Answer*_____

Correct Answers

A285

Answer 2 is correct. EENT-side effects and adverse reactions is tinnitus and/or hearing loss; 1) dry skin doesn't occur INTEG rash, urticaria, bruising; 3) CNS signs and symptoms are drowsiness, dizziness, confusion, convulsion, headache, flushing, hallucinations; 4) RESP signs and symptoms are wheezing hyperpnea.

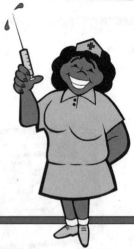

A286

Answer 1 is correct. Malaria is an infection caused by parasites. Infectious agents are plasmodium vivax, P. malariae, P. falciparum, and P. ovale; 2) poliomyelitis is an acute viral infection. The infectious agent is the polio virus (genus enterovirus). 3) Rabies is almost invariably a fatal acute viral encephalomyelitis if untreated. The infectious agent is the rabies virus, a rhabdovirus of the genus lyssavirus. 4) Yellow fever is an acute infectious viral disease of short duration and varying severity. The infectious agent is the virus of yellow fever, a flavivirus.

Questions

Q287

Mary Jones, a 29-year-old female, is admitted to the hospital, presenting with jaundice. The nurse assessing the patient would be aware that which of the following conditions may cause jaundice:

1) a deficiency in vitamin C
2) iron deficiency anemia
3) presence of the yeast spore
4) an obstruction in the common bile duct

*Your Own Answer*_____

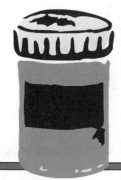

Q288

Mr. Jones was admitted to the burn unit with first degree burns. Which of the following would the nurse be least likely to observe:

1) mild to severe erythema
2) small thin-walled blisters
3) fat exposed
4) skin blanches with pressure

*Your Own Answer*_____

Correct Answers

A287

Answer 4 is correct. Obstruction in the common bile duct results in posthepatic jaundice caused by excessive production of bilirubin due to excessive red blood cell destruction; 1) vitamin C deficiency produces scurvy. Skin is rough and blotchy bruises appear, wounds fail to heal, blood and circulatory system produces pinpoint hemorrhages and atherosclerotic plaques; 2) iron deficiency anemia doesn't cause jaundice; 3) yeast spore doesn't cause jaundice.

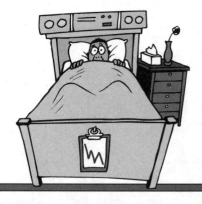

A288

Answer 3 is correct. Fat exposure occurs in third degree burns, which are also known as full thickness burns; 1) mild to severe erythema occurs with first degree burns. The burn only affects the epidermis. 2) Small thin-walled blisters occur in first degree burns, with only the epidermis involved; 4) skin blanches with pressure from first degree burns due to erythema and edema.

Questions

Q289

The nurse recognizes that the LEAST likely immediate treatment and first aid of a burn victim would be:

1) provide relief from pain
2) apply topical cream to newly-burned area
3) minimize contamination of wound
4) transport quickly

*Your Own Answer*_____

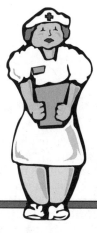

Q290

The nurse recognizes which of the following as generally considered to be a disease caused by a wound infection:

1) bacillary dysentery
2) gonorrhea
3) malaria
4) tetanus

*Your Own Answer*_____

Correct Answers

A289

Answer 2 is correct. Topical cream to newly burned area should never be applied. This activity is time-consuming as well as painful since the substance used will have to be removed for the physician to evaluate the wound. 1) and 3) can both be minimized by wrapping the affected area with a clean, moist towel or sheet. This decreases pain caused by air touching the exposed nerve ending. The covering also decreases the possibility of infection or contamination. 4) Rapid transport is essential to provide proper treatment and decrease loss of body heat from burn wounds.

A290

Answer 4 is correct. Tetanus is an acute disease induced by an exotoxin of the tetanus bacillus, which grows anaerobically at the site of an injury. 1) Bacillary dysentery is an acute bacterial disease caused by the genus shigella. Mode of transmission is by direct or indirect fecal-oral transmission from a patient or carrier. 2) Gonorrhea is a sexually-transmitted bacterial disease. Mode of transmission is by contact with exudates from mucous membranes of infected persons, almost always as a result of sexual activity. 3) Malaria is caused by parasites. The infectious agents are Plasmodium vivax, P. malariae, P. falciparum, and P. ovale.

Questions

c

Mr. Smith is brought into the emergency room with a diagnosis of barbiturate overdose. The nurse would expect to see the following signs and symptoms:

1) delirium and agitation
2) dilated pupils
3) constricted pupils
4) extrapyramidal tremor

*Your Own Answer*_____

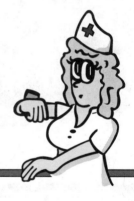

Q292

A physician orders a nurse to prepare Narcan 0.4 mg IM stat. The nurse would recognize that this antidote is commonly used for a substance overdose of:

1) deferoxamine
2) ethanol
3) narcotic and narcotic derivatives
4) oxygen

*Your Own Answer*_____

A291

Answer 1 is correct. Barbiturates are central nervous system depressants; 2) dilated pupils are seen with amphetamines; 3) constricted pupils are seen with morphine usage; 4) extra pyramidal tremors are seen with phenothiazines usage.

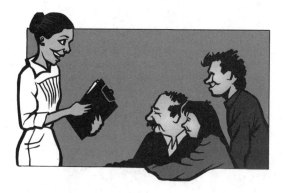

A292

Answer 3 is correct. Naloxone competes with narcotics at narcotic receptor sites; 1) deferoxamine is the antidote for iron, and it binds iron ions to form a water soluble complex that is removed by the kidneys; 2) ethanol is the antidote for the substance methanol; 4) oxygen is the antidote used for carbon monoxide overdose.

Questions

Q293

The nurse recognizes the person at highest risk of developing prostate cancer is:

1) 55-year-old black male
2) 45-year-old Caucasian male
3) 55-year-old Caucasian female
4) 45-year-old hispanic male

*Your Own Answer*_____

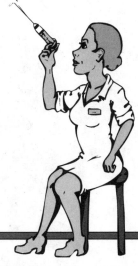

Q294

A patient with a history of subacute bacterial endocarditis is instructed by the physician to eliminate foods that act as cardiac stimulants. The nurse should instruct the patient to avoid:

1) chocolate
2) yogurt
3) red meats
4) club soda

*Your Own Answer*_____

Correct Answers

A293

Answer 1 is correct. Cancer of the prostate is rare before the age of 50, but increases with each decade. Black men develop it twice as frequently as Caucasian men and at an earlier age; 2) Caucasian men develop prostatic cancer half as frequently as black men, but more frequently than Hispanic men; 3) females are not physiologically capable of developing prostate cancer; 4) this group of men have a lower rate of prostate cancer than black and Caucasian males.

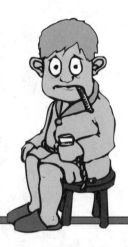

A294

Answer 1 is correct. Chocolate has a high caffeine content. It may stimulate catecholamine release and act as a cardiac stimulant; 2) yogurt doesn't act as a cardiac stimulant. It aids in digestion if lactose intolerance is present. 3) Red meats do not stimulate the myocardium; 4) club soda contains sodium chloride but does not stimulate the myocardium.

Questions

Q295

The medical-surgical nurse recognizes that a slowly progressive degenerative disease of the nervous system, usually occurring in or after middle life and characterized by tremors and rigidity of the skeletal muscles, is:

1) arthritis
2) Parkinson's disease
3) epilepsy
4) multiple sclerosis

*Your Own Answer*_____

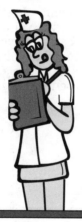

Q296

A positive sign of pregnancy is:

1) amenorrhea
2) uterine enlargement
3) Goodell's Sign
4) fetal heartbeat

*Your Own Answer*_____

Correct Answers

A295

Answer 2 is correct. Parkinson's disease is a slowly progressive degenerative process involving the basal ganglia and substantia nigra, which most often begins in the sixth decade of life. The three cardinal features are tremors, rigidity, and akinesia. 1) Arthritis occurs from childhood, depending on etiology. Pathological processes of arthritis affect the joint with inflammation and degenerative changes. 3) Epilepsy is a paroxysmal disorder of the nervous system that results in recurrent attacks of loss of consciousness or other types of seizures in which convulsion movements or other movement activity, sensory phenomena, or behavioral abnormalities may occur. Onset may occur at any age. 4) Multiple sclerosis is the most common cause of progressive neurologic disability in young adults in the U.S. as well as many other countries. A disorder characterized by multifocal areas of demyelination diffusely scattered throughout the central nervous system with a history of remissions and exacerbations, its onset happens between 20 and 40 years of age.

A296

Answer is 4. The fetal heartbeat is the only choice which directly involves the fetus, which is a positive sign of pregnancy. All other answer choices are probable indicators of pregnancy and could possibly be induced by other conditions.

Questions

Q297

One of the earliest signs of hypoxia is:

1) cyanosis
2) bradycardia
3) oliguria
4) restlessness

*Your Own Answer*_____

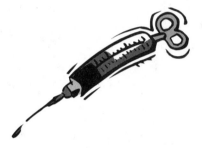

Q298

Mr. Smith is scheduled for surgery for a large bowel obstruction. You can assume that your pre-operative education has been successful if he states:

1) "I can have only breakfast on the morning of my surgery."
2) "I can resume eating food as soon as I fully wake up from the operation."
3) "I will be given nutrition intravenously so my bowel can start to heal."
4) "I can expect to have a lot of diarrhea."

*Your Own Answer*_____

Correct Answers

A297

Answer 4 is correct. Restlessness is an early cardinal sign of hypoxia. Cyanosis is a late sign of hypoxia. One would find a hypoxic person tachycardic, not bradycardic. Oliguria has no relation to hypoxia.

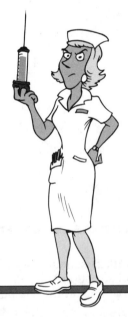

A298

Answer 3 is correct. A person undergoing bowel surgery would be required to be NPO at least after midnight on the night prior to the operation. Answer 2 is incorrect because the client would have to have the return of bowel sounds before he is allowed to eat or drink. Choice 4 is unrelated and should not be a factor.

Questions

Q299

A newborn is undergoing phototherapy for hyperbilirubinemia. Which of the following nursing interventions is not appropriate:

1) applying a shield to the infant's eyes
2) monitoring the body temperature
3) applying oil to the infant's skin
4) monitoring fluid intake and output

*Your Own Answer*_____

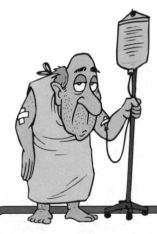

Q300

A patient is admitted to the hospital because of smoke inhalation and burns to the face from a grease fire. The nurse recognizes a life-threatening complication from this can be:

1) airway obstruction
2) cardiac arrest
3) body image disturbance
4) tension pneumothorax

*Your Own Answer*_____

Correct Answers

A299

Answer 3 is correct. All of the interventions are indicated except for applying oil to the infant's skin. This would potentially cause burns to the infant.

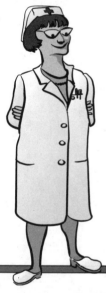

A300

Answer 1 is correct. An airway obstruction is a life-threatening complication that can occur especially with burns of the face and neck. Laryngeal edema develops, closing off the airway. While cardiac arrest is a life-threatening situation, it is not directly from the complication of burns. A body image disturbance is not life threatening. A tension pneumothorax is also not a relevant complication.

Questions

Q301

Mr. Jones has just been started on lithium for his long-standing depression. After two days of being on the medication, he complains that he still feels extremely sad. An appropriate response to Mr. Jones would be:

1) "I'll tell the doctor that you're still not feeling well."
2) "Maybe we need to increase your dosage."
3) "It may take one to two weeks before you actually start to feel better."
4) "You may be experiencing a temporary mood swing."

*Your Own Answer*_____

Q302

Mrs. Smith suddenly develops acute shortness of breath, with crackles throughout her lung fields. You obtain an order for Lasix 80mg IV Push. Shortly after diuresing a large amount of urine, Mrs. Smith complains of leg cramps. This is most likely attributed to:

1) lying in bed for a long period of time
2) poor circulation to her extremities
3) a low potassium level
4) hypoxia from the episode

*Your Own Answer*_____

Correct Answers

A301

Answer 3 is correct. Lithium levels usually peak shortly after administration of the dose. However, clinical effects may not be apparent for one to three weeks after the start of the drug. Informing Mr. Jones of this reduces his anxiety that he has not felt any better from the drug.

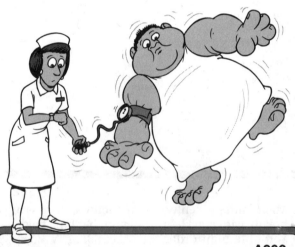

A302

Answer 3 is correct. Lasix is a loop diuretic that excretes potassium. Administration of a large amount of Lasix can quickly cause hypokalemia. A symptom of hypokalemia is muscle cramps.

Questions

Q303

Mr. Smith is admitted to the hospital with a diagnosis of new onset atrial fibrillation. His PR interval is noted to be:

1) between 0. 16-0.20 seconds
2) gradually lengthening before the QRS complex
3) greater than 0.20 seconds
4) unable to be determined

*Your Own Answer*_____

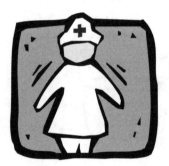

Q304

The appropriate sequencing of an abdominal examination includes:

1) inspection, percussion, ascultation, palpation
2) ascultation, inspection, palpation, percussion
3) inspection, ascultation, percussion, palpation
4) ascultation, inspection, percussion, palpation

*Your Own Answer*_____

Correct Answers

A303

Answer 4 is correct. Atrial fibrillation is characterized by a grossly irregular rhythm with unmeasurable PR interval. Answer 1 is a normal PR interval; answer 2 is seen in a Wenkebach rhythm; answer 3 is seen in a first degree AV block.

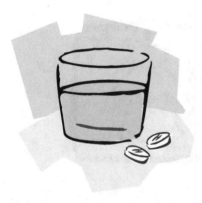

A304

Answer 3 is correct. Inspection is always the first fundamental portion of an exam. Ascultation is performed next in the sequence to ensure that bowel sounds have not been manipulated by percussion or palpation. Light and deep palpation are performed last.

Questions

Q305

Mrs. Jones, a client with chronic renal failure, complains of a tingling sensation around her mouth. The nurse elicits a positive Chvostek's sign. This indicates:

1) hypocalcemia
2) hypomagnesemia
3) hypercalcemia
4) hypermagnesemia

*Your Own Answer*_____

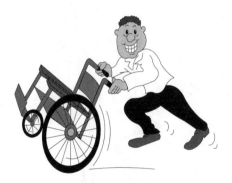

Q306

Acromegaly is a disorder related to the

1) adrenal glands
2) adrenal cortex
3) pituitary gland
4) parathyroid gland

*Your Own Answer*_____

Correct Answers

A305

Answer 1 is correct. Chvostek's sign is a twinge noted in the muscles of the face when the facial nerve is tapped below the zygomatic arch. This is an indicator of hypocalcemia, commonly seen in client's with renal failure.

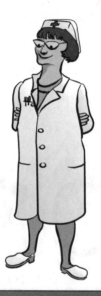

A306

Answer 3 is correct. Acromegaly is a disorder of excessive skeletal growth caused by a tumor of the pituitary gland. Surgical removal of the pituitary gland is often indicated for management of the disease.

Questions

Q307

A seventy-nine-year-old woman is bedridden and incontinent. It is noted on her chart that the client has a sacral decubitus ulcer involving the subcutaneous tissue with purulent drainage. This is characterized at which ulcer staging?

1) Stage I
2) Stage II
3) Stage III
4) Stage IV

*Your Own Answer*_____

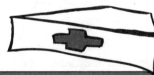

Q308

The nurse inserts a nasogastric tube for a client with severe abdominal pain. After the tube is inserted, the first action the nurse should take is:

1) irrigate the tube to determine patency
2) keep advancing the tube until resistance is met
3) fasten the tube securely to the client's face with adhesive tape
4) confirm placement of tube by ascultation

*Your Own Answer*_____

Correct Answers

A307

Answer 3 is correct. A Stage III decubitus ulcer ungluess the subcutaneous tissue and can have purulent drainage. Stage I indicates redness that blanches with pressure, but no skin breakdown. Stage II includes superficial skin breakdown with slight ulcer drainage. Stage IV is deep ulceration extending into the muscle or to the bone.

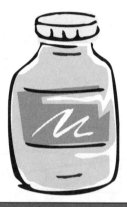

A308

Answer 4 is correct. The first action the nurse should take is to confirm placement. After the tube is verified as in the stomach, then it may be fastened to the client's nose with tape. 1) Irrigation should not be performed before verifying placement in case the tube is not in the stomach. 2) The tube should not be advanced further than the stomach, and should be measured prior to insertion.

Questions

Flail chest is characterized by:

1) tracheal deviation
2) paradoxical respiration
3) mediastinal flutter
4) oxygen toxicity

*Your Own Answer*_____

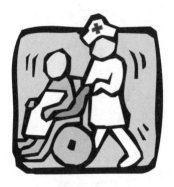

Q310

An abnormal finding of an abdominal assessment would be:

1) a firm liver edge at or above the costal margin
2) an unpalpable spleen
3) high pitched, gurgling bowel sounds
4) generalized rebound tenderness

*Your Own Answer*_____

Correct Answers

A309

Answer 2 is correct. Paradoxical respirations are seen in flail chest as the flail segment pulls inward during inspiration and bulges out during expiration. 1) Tracheal deviation is seen in a tension pneumothorax; 3) mediastinal flutter is seen in an open pneumothorax when the heart and large vessels are shifted during the respiratory cycle; 4) a low blood oxygen level usually accompanies flail chest.

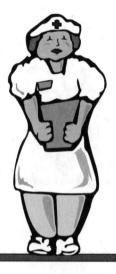

A310

Answer is 4. Rebound tenderness is always abnormal and may indicate peritoneal inflammation or perforation of an ulcer. Answers 1, 2, and 3 are all normal findings.

Questions

Q311

The nurse notices that a client's thyroid function studies indicate she has hypothyroidism. Which of the following is NOT an indication of hypothyroidism:

1) lethargy
2) muscular weakness
3) goiter
4) slow speech

*Your Own Answer*_____

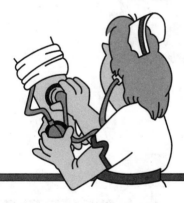

Q312

During the nursing admission health assessment, the nurse elicits from the client that he has difficulty initiating the flow of his urine. This is described as:

1) hesitancy
2) dysuria
3) dribbling
4) urgency

*Your Own Answer*_____

Correct Answers

A311

Answer 3 is correct. Goiter would be present in a client with hyperthyroidism. Answers 1, 2, and 4 are all symptoms of hypothyroidism.

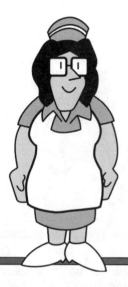

A312

Answer 1 is correct. Hesitancy is difficulty starting a stream of urine, which may be a symptom of obstruction or neurological dysfunction. 2) Dysuria is painful voiding. 3) Dribbling is the inability to control the passage of urine. 4) Urgency is the sudden need to void.

Questions

Q313

While ascultating a client's heart tones, the nurse notes an S3 heart sound. This sound is:

1) always abnormal in adults and children
2) the start of systole
3) heard often in clients with mitral regurgitation
4) heard often in clients with congestive heart failure

*Your Own Answer*_____

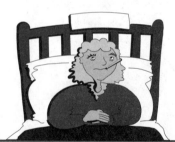

Q314

A client with a long-standing history of chronic obstructive pulmonary disease (COPD) presents to the nurse with crackles bilaterally in the lower lung fields and acute shortness of breath. A priority nursing diagnosis would be:

1) impaired gas exchange
2) ineffective airway clearance
3) altered tissue perfusion
4) activity intolerance

*Your Own Answer*_____

Correct Answers

A313

Answer 4 is correct. An S3 heart tone is a finding heard in clients with congestive heart failure. 1) An S3 heart tone may be normal in children. 2) An S1 heart tone marks the start of systole. 3) A murmur would be heard in mitral regurgitation.

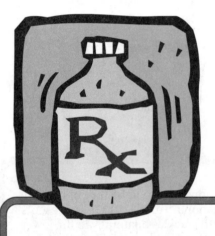

A314

Answer 1 is correct. Crackles hindering gas diffusion, combined with decreased compliance of the lung seen in COPD, make this a priority diagnosis. 2) This refers primarily to a decreased cough or gag reflex, or very thick secretions; 4) is an appropriate diagnosis, but not a priority.

Questions

Q315

A thirty-two-year-old client, a mother of two young children, is scheduled for a breast biopsy for a lump noted in her right breast on a routine physical exam. She says to the nurse, "I can't even imagine what I'll do if this is cancer." A therapeutic nursing response would be:

1) "Don't worry, I'm sure it won't be."
2) "If it is cancer, you can always have surgery."
3) "Tell me what you're most concerned about."
4) "Wait until the test results come back, then we will talk about it."

*Your Own Answer*_____

Q316

A forty-two-year-old man experiences an acute myocardial infarction. On his second hospital day, he develops an episode of substernal chest pain. He says to the nurse, "This wouldn't have happened if you people knew what you were doing." The client is using the defense mechanism of:

1) denial
2) rationalization
3) regression
4) displacement

*Your Own Answer*_____

Correct Answers

A315

Answer 3 is correct. Encourage the client to express fears and concerns. This fosters the development of coping mechanisms. 1) The nurse cannot assure this, therefore this would be detrimental. 2) This statement minimizes the client's feelings and closes discussion; 4) same as 2).

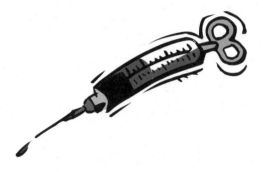

A316

Answer 4 is correct. Displacement transfers emotional feeling from the actual stressor, the client's condition, to a substitute, the hospital staff. 1) The client does not deny the pain exists; 2) he does not rationalize, or attribute it to another cause, i.e., heartburn; 3) the client does not pretend to be dependent or helpless.

Questions

Q317

The normal heart rate for a newborn is:

1) 120-170 beats per minute
2) 170-200 beats per minute
3) 80 -120 beats per minute
4) under 80 beats per minute

*Your Own Answer*_____

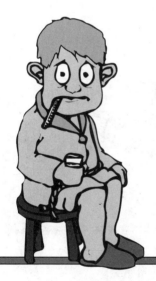

Q318

A nursing priority in the immediate postoperative period of an infant's cleft lip repair is to:

1) reassure the family of the gradual healing process
2) protect the operative site
3) prepare for discharge planning
4) cuddle the infant to prevent heat loss

*Your Own Answer*_____

Correct Answers

A317

Answer 1 is correct. The newborn's normal heart rate is between 120 and 170 beats per minute, with the average at about 130 beats per minute.

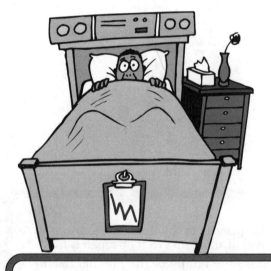

A318

Answer 2 is correct. Protecting the operative site is a priority so the site can stay clean and free of infection. Answer 1 is another function of the nurse, but not the priority; 3) can be started later in the hospitalization; 4) heat loss should not be a problem if the infant is properly swaddled.

Questions

Q319

A seven-year-old child shows the nurse her tongue; it is whitish, with a strawberry-like appearance. A few days later, the tongue is red strawberry. This a characteristic of which childhood disease:

1) rubella
2) mumps
3) poliomyelitis
4) scarlet fever

Your Own Answer

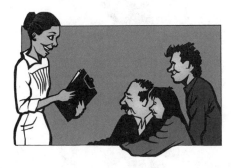

Q320

The nurse formulates a nursing care plan for an anorexic adolescent recently hospitalized. A priority nursing diagnosis for this client is:

1) body image disturbance
2) ineffective individual coping
3) altered nutrition; less than body requirements
4) self-care deficit: feeding

Your Own Answer

Correct Answers

A319

Answer 4 is correct. A white strawberry tongue occurs during the first two days of infection of scarlet fever. After the white sloughs off, the tongue becomes red and strawberry-like, about the fourth day. Answers 1, 2, and 3 do not exhibit these symptoms.

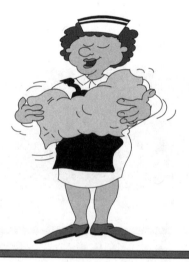

A320

Answer 3 is correct. This diagaosis would be a primary concern to an adolescent, whose nutrition would affect growth and development. Answers 1 and 2 are not priorities, but appropriate diagnoses. Answer 4, the client has no difficulty with feeding, but chooses not to feed self.

Questions

Q321

An anticipated emotional response of a woman who has just learned she is pregnant is:

1) denial
2) regression
3) frustration
4) ambivalence

Your Own Answer

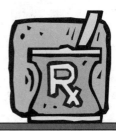

Q322

Your diabetic client requires insulin twice per day. Her usual regimen is eight units of regular insulin with ten units of neutral protamine Hagedorin (NPH) insulin. Before administering this, the nurse knows to:

1) use a five-milliliter syringe
2) use the last site used
3) substitute semilente for regular insulin
4) check for flocculation of the vials

Your Own Answer

Correct Answers

A321

Answer 4 is correct. Ambivalence is a common response women experience when they learn of their pregnancy. Often women have initial mixed feelings about motherhood. Answers 1 and 2 are not anticipated feelings. 3) Frustration is uncommon and not appropriate.

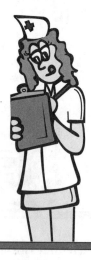

A322

Answer 4 is correct. Flocculation is clumping or a frosted appearance in the insulin. Regular insulin should be clear; NPH insulin should be milky white. 1) Insulin should be administered subcutaneously in a maximum of one milliliter syringe with unit delineations. 2) The sites for insulin administration should be rotated to foster absorption. 3) Semilente insulin action differs from regular insulin and therefore should not be substituted without a physician's order.

Questions

Q323

A young man is admitted with extensive burns caused by a fire at work. His electrocardiogram shows peaked T waves. The client denies chest pain, but does complain of severe pain of the lower extremities where the majority of the burns occurred. An initial expected electrolyte imbalance is:

1) hypomagnesemia
2) hyperkalemia
3) hypercalcemia
4) hypocalcemia

*Your Own Answer*_____

Q324

Mrs. Smith, a seventy-two-year-old client, underwent orthopedic surgery for a right hip fracture. Forty-eight hours after the surgery, she complains of calf pain. Lower extremity venous doppler studies are positive for a deep vein thrombosis. Soon after she arrives back in her room from the test, she develops an acute episode of shortness of breath. This may be attributed to:

1) pulmonary embolism
2) pulmonary edema
3) lobar pneumonia
4) anxiety disorder

*Your Own Answer*_____

Correct Answers

A323

Answer 2 is correct. After a burn injury, it is expected that the client will exhibit hyperkalemia due to the extensive cellular destruction, which releases potassium from the cell into the extracellular fluid. This can affect the client's electrocardiogram with peaked T waves.

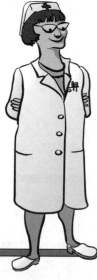

A324

Answer 1 is correct. After orthopedic surgery, elderly clients are predisposed to the development of a DVT. An episode of shortness of breath may indicate the clot became dislodged from the extremity landing in the pulmonary vasculature. This would need to be ruled out before any other disease process would become suspect.

Questions

Q325

An elderly gentleman is being evaluated for hearing loss in both ears. The nurse performs a Rinne test, which is negative. This means:

1) bone conduction of sound is greater than air conduction of sound
2) sound is heard equally in both ears
3) air conduction of sound is greater than bone conduction
4) whispers are heard easily in both ears

*Your Own Answer*_____

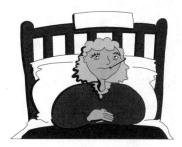

Q326

When testing the cranial nerves III, IV, and VI, the nurse may ask the client to:

1) open his mouth and say "ah"
2) move his eyes through different visual fields
3) shrug his shoulders against resistance
4) wrinkle his forehead and smile

*Your Own Answer*_____

Correct Answers

A325

Answer 1 is correct. A Rinne test evaluates the ability to detect bone conduction versus air conduction of sound. If air conduction is greater, then the Rinne test is positive, which is a normal finding. If bone conduction is greater, this is Rinne negative and it indicates hearing loss.

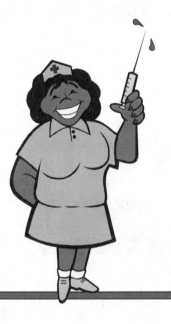

A326

Answer 2 is correct. The oculomotor, trochlear, and abducens cranial nerves involve extraocular movements. Answer 1 would test the vagus cranial nerve; answer 3 would test the spinal accessory cranial nerve; and answer 4 tests the facial cranial nerve.

Questions

Q327

The parents of a two-year-old boy bring him to a pediatric clinic to be evaluated. The parents state the child has been unusually hyperactive over the last few days. They report the child may be acting out since they have been concentrating on refinishing their house, and may not have been paying enough attention to the child. The nurse knows this child should be screened for:

1) physical abuse
2) acetaminophen poisoning
3) lead poisoning
4) attention deficit disorder

*Your Own Answer*_____

Q328

A client known to have a history of diabetes was brought in from the nursing home and diagnosed with diabetic ketoacidosis. The nurse notes the client has a fruity odor to his breath. She also observes which type of respirations that would counteract acidosis:

1) Cheyne-Stokes respirations
2) Kussmaul respirations
3) Hypoventilatory respirations
4) Parodoxical respirations

*Your Own Answer*_____

Correct Answers

A327

Answer 3 is correct. Lead poisoning commonly occurs in children between the ages of nine months and six years, when children are more apt to place objects inside of their mouths. Hyperactivity is a symptom of lead poisoning, also refinishing the house may expose the child to paint containing lead. 1) There is no evidence to indicate physical abuse. 2) Acetaminophen poisoning is not characterized by hyperactivity. 4) ADD does not develop suddenly.

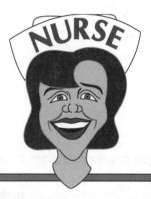

A328

Answer 2 is correct. Kussmaul respirations are marked by an increase in depth and respiratory rate. These act to compensate for acidosis by blowing off carbon dioxide, thus raising the pH of the blood. 1) Cheyne-Stokes respirations are seen with a depression of the respiratory center or in heart failure. Answer 3 would increase acidosis by the retention of carbon dioxide, and answer 4 would not counteract acidosis.

Questions

Q329

A client with metastatic colon cancer has been placed on neutropenic precautions. The nurse places a sign indicating this outside the client's room. Another appropriate nursing action is:

1) instruct family members that the client is now on strict isolation
2) restrict the client's activity level to bed rest for twenty-four hours
3) ensure that fresh fruits and vegetables are not on client's meal trays
4) offer an antiemetic around the clock for anticipated nausea

*Your Own Answer*_____

Q330

The nurse is preparing a thirty-five-year-old pregnant woman for an emergency delivery for abruptio placentae. As the client is prepped, the nurse notes several areas of petechiae on the client's hand and a large ecchymotic area on her left forearm where blood had been drawn. Her blood pressure in the right arm is 104/70. This client may be developing:

1) impending eclampsia
2) uterine rupture
3) superficial thromboembolism
4) disseminated intravascular coagulation

*Your Own Answer*_____

Correct Answers

A329

Answer 3 is correct. Neutropenia indicates a client's decreased ability to fight infection, manifested by an abnormally low white blood cell count. The client should avoid fresh fruits and vegetables because they harbor bacteria, even after cleansing. 1) The client would not require isolation. 2) Strict bed rest is not necessary. 4) Nausea is not related to neutropenia.

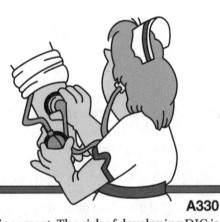

A330

Answer 4 is correct. The risk of developing DIC is increased in the setting of abruptio placentae. Early signs of DIC include petechiae and ecchymosis. 1) Hypertension would be seen in eclampsia. 2) Severe abdominal pain and the onset of shock would be seen in uterine rupture. 3) No evidence of thromboembolism is present.

Questions

Q331

A client with liver failure has been intermittently confused and unable to coordinate his hands to eat. The physician prescribes a regimen of lactulose (Cephulac) twice per day. The nurse knows this is given to decrease which of the following blood levels:

1) ammonia
2) potassium
3) urea
4) creatinine

*Your Own Answer*_____

Q332

Mrs. Edwards is an insulin-dependent diabetic. She has been placed on frequent blood sugar fingerstick checks to try to determine the reason for her persistent morning hyperglycemia. Her blood sugar at bedtime is 182. At three a.m., her blood sugar is 67. At seven a.m., her blood sugar is 284. This pattern is suggestive of:

1) dawn phenomenon
2) insulin waning
3) Somogyi Effect
4) hyperinsulinism

*Your Own Answer*_____

Correct Answers

A331

Answer 1 is correct. Ammonia builds up in the blood when the liver cells are unable to convert it to urea for excretion. As ammonia accumulates in the bloodstream, neurological impairment is observed, affecting mental status and coordination. Lactulose acts to trap ammonia in the colon and promote its excretion through stool.

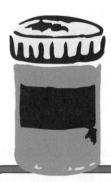

A332

Answer 3 is correct. The Somogyi Effect is characterized by a normal or elevated blood sugar at bedtime, followed by hypoglycemia during the early morning hours leading to a rebound hyperglycemia by morning. 1) Dawn's Phenomenon shows normal blood sugar levels until about three a.m. when levels gradually start to rise. 2) Insulin waning is the gradual rise of blood sugar levels throughout the night. 4) No elevations in blood sugar would be seen in hyperinsulinism.

Questions

The nurse is caring for a twenty-four-year-old male who fractured his femur during a football game. The client has become increasingly irritable and restless, frequently calling for the nurse and ringing the call bell. An appropriate nursing action is:

1) provide diversional activities to control the client's irritability
2) reassure the client that it is normal to feel restricted because of his fracture
3) medicate the client more frequently for breakthrough pain
4) call the physician and notify him or her of the client's behavior

*Your Own Answer*_____

An infant with an intact myelomeningocele is being prepared for surgery. The nurse assesses the infant and does not:

1) put a moist, sterile, and nonsticking dressing over the myelomeningocele
2) keep the infant in a prone position
3) apply a high absorbency diaper
4) measure the infant's head circumference

*Your Own Answer*_____

Correct Answers

A333

Answer 4 is correct. The physician should be notified immediately of any neurological changes, especially if seen in the setting of a long bone fracture. This may be an early symptom of a fat embolism, which would need immediate evaluation. Answers 1, 2, and 3 all neglect to realize the potential of a fat embolism.

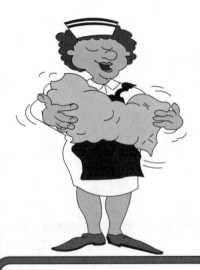

A334

Answer 3 is correct. Applying a diaper is contraindicated for an infant with a myelomeningocele until well after the surgery when the healing process has begun. Answer 1 is appropriate to prevent infection. Answer 2 is also appropriate to minimize trauma and tension. Answer 4 is necessary to observe for hydocephalus.

Questions

Q335

An eighty-year-old man was admitted following an acute cerebrovascular accident (CVA). The client has mild weakness on the right side of his body, along with an expressive aphasia. After several attempts to communicate with the nurse, the client becomes frustrated, and refuses any further attempts at verbal communication. Which of the following is least appropriate:

1) reduce the environmental noise
2) alter speech patterns to a child's level
3) provide alternate methods of communication
4) use "yes" or "no" questions

*Your Own Answer*_____

Q336

A client with end stage renal disease returns from the operating room after placement of a Tankoff catheter. The nurse initiates peritoneal dialysis that evening. During the dwell time of the first exchange, the client complains of mild shortness of breath. The first intervention the nurse makes is to:

1) change the client's position in bed
2) apply oxygen at two liters per minute by nasal cannula
3) stop the dialysis treatment and call the physician
4) immediately drain the dialysate from the client

*Your Own Answer*_____

Correct Answers

A335

Answer 2 is correct. The client with expressive aphasia has difficulty in expressing his thoughts and words. He has no difficulty in understanding speech and content, as in receptive aphasia. Therefore, talking to the client like a child would only aggravate the client's frustration and may be insulting.

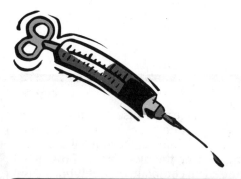

A336

Answer 1 is correct. Clients having peritoneal dialysis may experience shortness of breath caused by the instilled fluid pressing against the diaphragm. Usually this can be relieved by altering the client's position to even the distribution of fluid in the peritoneal cavity. Answers 2, 3, and 4 would not be the first intervention.

Questions

Q337

A sixty-five-year-old male with a history of alcohol abuse and coronary artery disease is admitted for bleeding esophageal varices. The physician prescribes an intravenous drip of Vasopressin (Pitressin). This client must be carefully monitored for the development of:

1) duodenal ulcer
2) pulmonary embolism
3) angina pectoris
4) acute renal failure

*Your Own Answer*_____

Q338

A client with newly-diagnosed Parkinson's disease has been taking Levodopa for relief of his symptoms. Recently his family has noticed that the client has been making weird facial expressions and noises with his mouth. The client's family should be informed that:

1) the client may be experiencing a toxicity of the drug
2) the client is having a normal response to the drug called a bradykinesia
3) the appearance of these types of symptoms indicates the disease may be getting better
4) the client is experiencing some common side effects of the drug

*Your Own Answer*_____

Correct Answers

Answer 3 is correct. Because Vasopressin can constrict the coronary arteries, the client's history of CAD predisposes him to angina, which may lead to myocardial infarction. Answers 1, 2, and 4 are not potential complications.

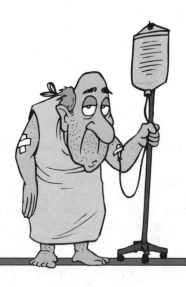

Answer 4 is correct. Facial grimacing and lip smacking movements are called dyskinesias, or abnormal involuntary movements, which are common side effects of Levodopa therapy.

Questions

Q339

A thirty-three-year-old woman is being evaluated by a physician for complaints of fatigue and weakness. The physician orders an injection of Tensilon (edrophonium). After the nurse gives the injection, the client's strength improves dramatically for a short time only. This client is suffering from which of the following disorders:

1) myasthenia gravis
2) Huntington's Disease
3) muscular dystrophy
4) multiple sclerosis

*Your Own Answer*_____

Q340

The nurse observes an abnormally low serum sodium level in the client with oat cell carcinoma of the lung. Upon further investigation, the nurse notes an increased urinary sodium, and a ten pound weight gain of the client in two days. The nurse reports these findings to the physician and suspects the client is experiencing:

1) acute tubular necrosis
2) syndrome of inappropriate antidiuretic hormone
3) nephrotic, syndrome
4) diabetes insipidus

*Your Own Answer*_____

Correct Answers

A339

Answer 1 is correct. Myasthenia gravis is a disorder of the transmission of nerve impulses to the muscles. Tensilon facilitates this transmission, therefore the improvement of symptoms confirms this diagnosis.

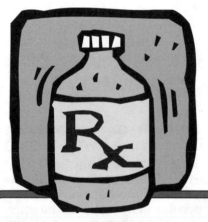

A340

Answer 2 is correct. SIADH is seen as a complication in clients with carcinomas of the lung; cells excrete ADH causing the disorder. A dilutional hyponatremia is caused by increased fluid volume, which would cause weight gain. Consequently, the body attempts to compensate and rid the body of the excess volume by excreting sodium.

Questions

A fifty-four-year-old man diagnosed with acute pancreatitis has severe abdominal pain. He says to the nurse, "Give me morphine. I've had it in the past and I know it works." The nurse should:

1) prepare to get a doctor's order for a small dose of morphine
2) not administer the morphine because of its addictive properties
3) not administer the morphine because of its contraindication in pancreatitis
4) administer the morphine and carefully monitor the client for hypotension

*Your Own Answer*_____

The daughter of a sixty-five-year-old woman brings her mother to the hospital because of confusion and headaches. The nurse elicits a positive Kernig's sign. Kernig's sign indicates:

1) increased intracranial pressure
2) cerebral vasospasm
3) meningeal irritation
4) cerebral edema

*Your Own Answer*_____

Correct Answers

A341

Answer 3 is correct. Morphine is contraindicated in clients with pancreatitis because it causes spasms in the sphincter of Oddi. Demerol (Meperidine) would be an appropriate medication to administer.

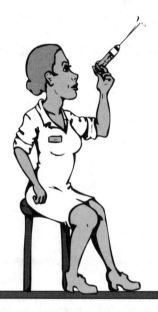

A342

Answer 3 is correct. Kernig's sign is positive when the client cannot fully extend her leg when lying with her thigh flexed on the abdomen. This is a sign of meningeal irritation and possibly meningitis.

Questions

A five-year-old child has been in the hospital for the past six days with acute poststreptococcal glomerulonephritis. The child's mother has been staying at the hospital since the admission. She approaches the nurse by stating, "Johnny has been urinating a lot more since last night. Is this normal?" The nurse should respond by stating:

1) "It may be a sign that his kidneys are weakening."
2) "It does not indicate any change in his status."
3) "It's not normal, I will notify the physician."
4) "It is usually the first sign of improvement."

*Your Own Answer*_____

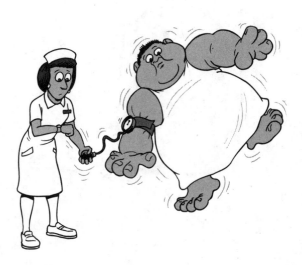

Correct Answers

A343

Answer 4 is correct. An increase in urine output will be the first indication of improvement in a child with glomerulonephritis. The mother should also be told to anticipate continued diuresis over the next two days, with a subsequent report of feeling better from her child. Answers 1, 2, and 3 are false.

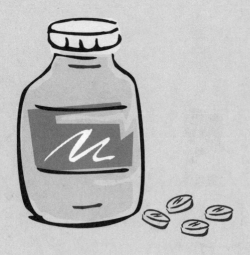

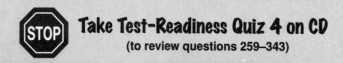

STOP **Take Test-Readiness Quiz 4 on CD**
(to review questions 259–343)

INDEX

Fluid balance
  assessment of, 156
  and jugular venous distention, 163
  and lung sounds, 156, 158
  organs and glands involved in, 32
  and orthostatic hypotension, 160
  postoperative, 47, 210
Fluoxetine, initial dosage of, 5
Focusing technique in client stress, 261
Food. *See also* Nutrition
  allergic reactions to, 113
  as cardiac stimulant, 294
  potassium content of, 266
  precautions in neutropenia, 329
  protein content of, in pregnancy, 86
Foot care in diabetes mellitus, 257
Fractures
  cast application in, 248
  fat embolism in, 333
  of hip, deep vein thrombosis in, 229, 324
Furosemide therapy
  hypokalemia in, 302
  onset and duration of action in, 283
Gallstones in elderly, nonsurgical management of, 132
Gases, arterial blood, 31
  in respiratory acidosis, 28
  in respiratory alkalosis, 30
Glomerulonephritis, urinary output in, 343
Glove use, 55
  disposal of gloves after, 167
Glucose blood levels
  in chronic hyperglycemia, 152
  management strategies on, 155
  in Somogyi effect, 332
  and symptoms in hypoglycemia, 150, 252
  in type II diabetes mellitus, 151
Glucose tolerance test, indications for, 153, 154

Group therapy
  in alcohol abuse, 137
  in psychiatric unit, 12
Hallucinations in schizophrenia, 13, 16, 136
Handwashing, 55
Hearing aid use, preoperative preparations in, 185
Hearing loss
  in aspirin overdose, 285
  Rinne test in, 325
Heart failure
  central venous pressure monitoring in, 162
  heart sounds in, 313
  jugular venous distention in, 163
  nutrition in, 123
  weight measurements in, 270
Heart rate of newborn, 317
Heart sounds in heart failure, 313
Hemolytic anemia, 281
Hemorrhage
  in cardiac catheterization, signs of, 102
  in esophageal varices, 108, 337
  postoperative, 219-221
    hypovolemic shock in, 40, 219
    shunting of blood in, 220
    volume of blood loss in, 221
Heparin therapy
  in deep vein thrombosis, 239
  in pulmonary embolism, 241
Hernia, hiatal, 121
Herpes genitalis infection, 260
Hiatal hernia, 121
Hiccoughs, 245
Hip
  dysplasia of, congenital, 100
  fractures of, deep vein thrombosis in, 229, 324
HIV infection and AIDS, 25, 26
Homans sign in deep vein thrombosis, 236
Home care
  first visit by nurse in, 275
  in nasogastric intubation, 70

anaphylactic reactions to foods in, 113
in diabetes mellitus, 27, 155
and hypoglycemia, 150, 151
in endocarditis history, 294
in gallstones of elderly, 132
in heart failure, 123
in hypertension, 142
sodium restriction in, 253, 269
in neutropenia precautions, 329
parenteral, goals of, 183
potassium sources in, 266
in pregnancy, 84-86
preoperative, 181, 182, 298
and postoperative wound healing, 182
in urinary tract infections, 58
Obesity, laboratory screening tests in, 153
Opiates
naloxone reversal of, 206, 264, 292
in sickle cell crisis, 99
Ortolani's sign in congenital hip dysplasia, 100
Osteoporosis, drug therapy in, 127
Overdose. *See* Toxic conditions
Oxygen therapy
in COPD, 111, 203
in suctioning process, 205
Pain medications, 179, 180
naloxone reversal of, 206, 264, 292
in pancreatitis, 341
in sickle cell crisis, 99
underuse of, 99, 180
Pancreatitis, pain medications in, 341
Papilloma, 284
Parents
of chronically ill child, stress and anxiety of, 94
of neonate, adaptive behavior of, 80
Parkinson's disease, 295
levodopa therapy in, 338
pH of blood in respiratory acidosis, 28

Pharyngitis, streptococcal, antibiotic therapy in, 135
Photosensitivity from antibiotic therapy in cystitis, 109
Phototherapy in hyperbilirubinemia of neonate, 299
Phrenic nerve in hiccoughs, 245
Pine nut allergy, 113
Pituitary disorders, acromegaly in, 306
Placenta
abruption of, 330
previa, 87
Plaquenil sulfate therapy, instructions on, 249
Pneumococcal vaccine, 145
Pneumonia
contraindication to surgery in, 170
pneumococcal, prevention of, 145
postoperative, 218
signs and symptoms in, 279
Polycythemia vera, signs and symptoms in, 282
Positioning of clients
after needle biopsy of liver, 101
in breathing exercises, postoperative, 176
for comfort, postoperative, 45
in dialysis, 336
in grand mal seizure, 112
in hypovolemic shock, 224
in pulmonary embolism, 243
for skin care in immobility, 115, 259
for sleeping during pregnancy, 71
Postmenopausal women, symptoms and concerns in, 82
Postoperative period
in alcohol abuse history, 168
atelectasis in, 39, 204, 216, 217
blood pressure in, 201, 212, 267
blood tests in, 209
body image alterations in, 22, 66

and postoperative wound healing, 182
in pneumonia, 170
removal of nail polish and makeup in, 184
in renal disorders, 165
safety concerns in, 188
in tonsillectomy of child, 93
Pressure sores, 115, 259, 307
Prostate cancer risk, 293
Protein intake in pregnancy, 86
Psychiatric disorders
admission interview in, 8
assessment in community clinic, 10
bipolar disorder, 11
depression. *See* Depression
group therapy in, 12
schizophrenia, 13, 16, 136
suicidal behavior in, 1-3
therapeutic relationship in, 9
Pulse rate, 157
Pyelonephritis, symptoms in, 133
Radial pulse, 157
Rales in fluid volume overload, 158
Rationalization, definition of, 17
Rebound tenderness in abdominal examination, 310
Recovery room
hypotension in, 201
immediate assessment procedures in, 197, 198
release criteria in, 49
reorientation to time and place in, 214
return of sensory functions in, 199
Reflexes, in recovery from anesthesia, 196, 202
Repression, as defense mechanism, 263
Respiratory disorders
anesthesia and surgery in, 159
contraindication in pneumonia, 170

preoperative preparations in, 164
in burns and smoke inhalation, 300
chronic obstructive. *See* COPD
in flail chest, 309
pneumonia. *See* Pneumonia
postoperative
atelectasis, 39, 204, 216, 217
breathing exercises in, 116, 173-176, 204
cough techniques in, 116, 177
immediate assessment of, 197, 198, 200
incentive spirometry in, 173-175
naloxone reversal of opiates in, 206
prevention of, 48, 116, 178
procedures with risk for, 215
signs of, 200
splinting of incision in, 116, 177
ventilatory support in, 208
in tuberculosis, 143
Retinopathy, diabetic, 130
Rheumatoid arthritis
physical examination in, 246
treatment goals in, 247
Rhinitis, allergic, 134
Rinne test in hearing loss, 325
Rubella vaccination, postpartum, 77
Safety concerns
in depression, 1, 4
in falls of elderly, 106
in preoperative preparations, 188
in storage of medications
at bedside, 38, 105
of controlled substances, 271
in visitor monitoring and restriction
in depressed client, 4
in young trauma patient, 104
Scarlet fever, tongue appearance in, 319

Schizophrenia, 13
    hallucinations in, 13, 16, 136
Scoliosis screening, 258
Screening procedures
    in diabetes mellitus, 153, 154
    for scoliosis, 258
Seizures
    grand mal, 112
    in preeclampsia and eclampsia,
        88-90
Sensory functions in recovery from
    anesthesia, 199
Septic shock, 225-227
    early signs of, 41, 226
    in nosocomial infections, 225,
        227
    organisms causing, 223, 225
    prevention of, 227
    priority interventions in, 41
Septicemia
    antibiotic therapy in, 230
    in nosocomial infections, 225
Sexual abuse, 18
Sexually transmitted diseases
    contraceptive methods in
        prevention of, 120
    herpes genitalis in, 260
Shivering, postoperative, 207
Shock
    hypovolemic, 40, 219, 222, 224
    septic, 41, 223, 225-227
Shunting of blood, postoperative
    in atelectasis, 217
    in hemorrhage, 220
Sickle cell anemia, 98
    pain management in crisis, 99
Sinusitis, signs and symptoms in,
    134
Skin care
    in immobility, 115, 259
    in sun exposure, 124
Skin test in tuberculosis, 143
Sleeping position in pregnancy, 71
Smoke inhalation in burns, 300
Sodium intake in hypertension,
    253, 269

Somogyi effect, 332
Spirometry, incentive, 173-175
    coordination with meal time,
        174, 175
    indications for, 173
    nausea in, 174, 175
Splinting of incision for postopera-
    tive cough, 116, 177
Sterile technique, indications for, 56
Storage of medications
    at bedside, safety concerns in,
        38, 105
    of controlled substances, 271
    temperature requirements in, 272
Streptococcal infections
    pharyngitis in, 135
    pneumococcal vaccine against,
        145
Streptokinase in pulmonary
    embolism, contraindication to,
    244
Stress and anxiety
    focusing technique in, 261
    of newly admitted patient, 103
    of parents with chronically ill
        child, 94
    of recovering alcoholic, coping
        strategies in, 138
    repression as defense mecha-
        nism in, 263
Succinylcholine, respiratory
    depression from, 208
Suctioning process, oxygen therapy
    in, 205
Suicidal behavior, 1-3
Sulfamethoxazole and
    trimethoprim in cystitis,
    photosensitivity from, 109
Sun exposure
    prevention of skin cancer in, 124
    sensitivity to, in antibiotic
        therapy for cystitis, 109
Surgery
    anesthesia recovery in. *See*
        Anesthesia recovery
    aseptic technique in, 56

Notes

Notes

The ESSENTIALS®
of MATH & SCIENCE

Each book in the ESSENTIALS series offers all essential information of the field it covers. It summarizes what every textbook in the particular field must include, and is designed to help students in preparing for exams and doing homework. The ESSENTIALS are excellent supplements to any class text.

The ESSENTIALS are complete and concise with quick access to needed information. They serve as a handy reference source at all times. The ESSENTIALS are prepared with REA's customary concern for high professional quality and student needs.

Available in the following titles:

Advanced Calculus
Algebra & Trigonometry I & II
Anatomy & Physiology
Astronomy
Automatic Control Systems /
    Robotics
Biochemistry
Biology I & II
Biology of the Universe
Boolean Algebra
Calculus I, II & III
Chemistry
Complex Variables I & II
Computer Science I & II
Data Structures I & II
Differential Equations

Electric Circuits
Electromagnetics I & II
Electronic Communications II
Electronics I & II
Fluid Mechanics / Dynamics I
Genetics: Unlocking the
    Mysteries of Life
Geometry I & II
Group Theory I & II
Heat Transfer II
LaPlace Transforms
Linear Algebra
Math for Computer Applications
Math for Engineers II
Mechanics I, II & III
Microbiology

Modern Algebra
Numerical Analysis I & II
Organic Chemistry I & II
Physical Chemistry II
Physics I & II
Pre-Calculus
Probability
Real Variables
Set Theory
Statistics I & II
Strength of Materials &
    Mechanics of Solids II
Thermodynamics II
Topology
Transport Phenomena I & II

If you would like more information about any of these books,
complete the coupon below and return it to us or visit your local bookstore.

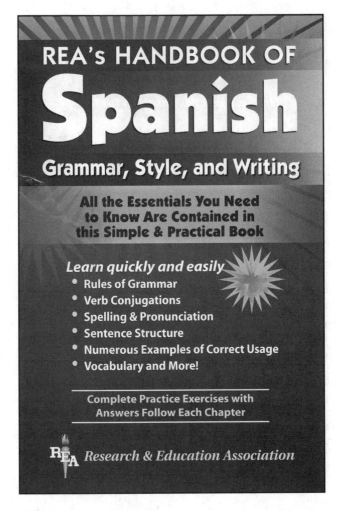

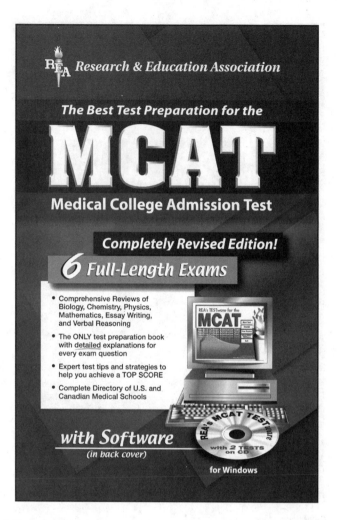

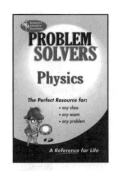

REA's **Test Preps**
The Best in Test Preparation

- REA "Test Preps" are **far more** comprehensive than any other test preparation series
- Each book contains up to **eight** full-length practice tests based on the most recent exams
- **Every** type of question likely to be given on the exams is included
- Answers are accompanied by **full** and **detailed** explanations

REA publishes over 70 Test Preparation volumes in several series. They include:

Advanced Placement Exams (APs)
Biology
Calculus AB & Calculus BC
Chemistry
Economics
English Language & Composition
English Literature & Composition
European History
French
Government & Politics
Physics B & C
Psychology
Spanish Language
Statistics
United States History
World History

College-Level Examination Program (CLEP)
Analyzing and Interpreting Literature
College Algebra
Freshman College Composition
General Examinations
General Examinations Review
History of the United States I
History of the United States II
Human Growth and Development
Introductory Sociology
Principles of Marketing
Spanish

SAT Subject Tests
Biology E/M
Chemistry
English Language Proficiency Test
French
German

SAT Subject Tests (cont'd)
Literature
Mathematics Level 1, 2
Physics
Spanish
United States History

Graduate Record Exams (GREs)
Biology
Chemistry
Computer Science
General
Literature in English
Mathematics
Physics
Psychology

ACT - ACT Assessment

ASVAB - Armed Services Vocational Aptitude Battery

CBEST - California Basic Educational Skills Test

CDL - Commercial Driver License Exam

CLAST - College Level Academic Skills Test

COOP & HSPT - Catholic High School Admission Tests

ELM - California State University Entry Level Mathematics Exam

FE (EIT) - Fundamentals of Engineering Exams - For both AM & PM Exams

FTCE - Florida Teacher Certification Exam

GED - High School Equivalency Diploma Exam (U.S. & Canadian editions)

GMAT - Graduate Management Admission Test

LSAT - Law School Admission Test

MAT - Miller Analogies Test

MCAT - Medical College Admission Test

MTEL - Massachusetts Tests for Educator Licensure

NJ HSPA - New Jersey High School Proficiency Assessment

NYSTCE: LAST & ATS-W - New York State Teacher Certification

PLT - Principles of Learning & Teaching Tests

PPST - Pre-Professional Skills Tests

PSAT / NMSQT

SAT

TExES - Texas Examinations of Educator Standards

THEA - Texas Higher Education Assessment

TOEFL - Test of English as a Foreign Language

TOEIC - Test of English for International Communication

USMLE Steps 1,2,3 - U.S. Medical Licensing Exams

U.S. Postal Exams 460 & 470

Research & Education Association
61 Ethel Road W., Piscataway, NJ 08854
Phone: (732) 819-8880   **website: www.rea.com**

Please send me more information about your Test Prep books.

Name _____

Address _____

City _____ State _____ Zip _____